Movement Is Life

A Holistic Approach to Exercise for Older Adults

Movement Is Life

A Holistic Approach to Exercise for Older Adults

Eva Desca Garnet

PRINCETON BOOK COMPANY, *Publishers*
PRINCETON, NEW JERSEY

Movement is Life: A Holistic Approach to Exercise for Older Adults is the textbook component of the three-part *Movement is Life* materials. The other components are: four double-track cassette tapes (1) *Invitation to Exercise / The Basic Lesson,* (2) *Once More - With Feeling / Once More - With Understanding,* (3) *Think With Your Body / Feel With Your Mind,* (4) *Rhythm and Rhyme in Country Dance Time / Chair Skwairs;* and *Chair Exercise Manual* which contains the complete, follow-along tapescripts, illustrations, and lesson plans. All of these materials may be ordered from Princeton Book Company, Publishers, P.O. Box 109, Princeton, New Jersey 08540.

Acknowledgments

I WISH TO EXPRESS my gratitude to the many people whose interest and expertise made this project possible:

to the administrators in the public and private sectors who originally supported the pioneering concept of a geriatric body dynamics program: Eva Van Skivers, Social Welfare Department of California; William Heideman, California Association of Homes for the Aging; Edward Denny, U.S. Department of Labor, Bureau of Apprenticeship and Training; Sergei Nutkiewitz, Westside Jewish Community Center, Los Angeles; Arthur N. Schwartz, Ph.D., University of Southern California;

and to those who later gave much appreciated support: Forrest Dillon, Rosemead Adult School; Alma Hawkins, PH.D., Dance Department, University of California, Los Angeles;

to the administrators, directors, and participants who permitted the photographic illustrations to be taken in their convalescent hospitals, retirement homes, and senior citizen centers: Lilly Telles, El Monte Convalescent Hospital; James R. Bennett, California Christian Home; Pastor Gilbert Moore, Solheim Lutheran Home; Mildred Garcia, Sun Ray East Convalescent Hospital; Ralph Jordan, Beverlywood Senior Citizen Center; Miriam Ludwig, Southern California Joint Board, Amalgamated Clothing Workers Union;

to the geriatricians who graciously shared their time and enthusiasm for my work both privately and publicly: Jack Agins, M.D.; Miquel Drobinsky, M.D.; and to Alvin I. Goldfarb, M.D., Geriatric Service, Mount Sinai Hospital, N.Y.C., for permission to reproduce "Components of Disorder: Psychodynamic Sequence;"

to my long-time friends and advisors: Genieve Fox, who opened windows in my inner world and doors in the outer world; Edith Perlmutter, Ph.D., for invaluable feedback and proofreading; Sara Kahn, co-worker during the early years of the project; and to Miriam Sherman, for periodic prodding; Linda Fichman, for periodic

Acknowledgments

brainstorming; Polly Dye and Mildred Bobo, for responding to the program with geriatric insight; Kathryn Keller, for assistance with research and proofreading;

to typist friends who rescued meaning out of scribble: Eleanor Randall, Janet Brown, Geri Stone, Ursula Kodas, Tamara Comstock;

to all my teachers, colleagues, and students who shared their movement experiences and insights with me;

to my special editor, Sally Cerny, and publisher, Charles H. Woodford, who helped evolve a viable structure for the multi-sensory approach of the text;

to my loving family, Leo, Janis, and Polly, I am especially grateful for their understanding and affection during the stressful years of the evolvement and completion of this project.

E.D.G.

Foreword

I HAVE WRITTEN this book out of concern for the well–being of the more than 23 million elderly people in our country, and for the rest of us, as well, in the hope that we may enjoy the use of our full potential in later years.

Experience with my mother's aging first inspired me to learn all I could of the aging process and to find ways to enrich life for older people. What I had to offer, as I saw it, was to return the gift of movement to older people, teaching them to make their days a life-filled time, so that their lives might be truly *lived* to the end.

But movement is more than a gift. It is a birthright—it is *life itself.* This realization has deepened as year after year I have seen old people who had surrendered to immobility, change. Transformed through movement, they become alert, responsive men and women who enjoy their increased vitality.

During the 20 years I have been working with older people, I have daily responded to their innermost feelings. They have expressed their pleasure and their pain. Some days the pleasure outweighs the pain. At other times, preoccupation with dissatisfaction leaps to the fore. At any age, we proclaim these states of mind as "good days" and "bad days." Our sense of contentment, and even happiness, depends on which outnumbers the other. Also, I have observed that the bad days are frequently the result of lack of freedom of action or of choice.

The years of teaching classes in adult education, recreation, and movement therapy at various institutions, including retirement homes, convalescent homes, convalescent hospitals and sanitaria, community centers, senior citizen centers, and parks have given substance to my belief that movement is the fundamental condition essential to aging successfully.

I am indebted to the thousands of older people with whom I

Foreword

have worked. They have helped shape my ideas through their enthusiasm, criticism, information, and the transforming response of their bodies.

For the theoretical foundation on which the concepts of this book rest, I have leaned heavily upon the humanist and physiological psychologists, social gerontologists, and geriatricians. The movement techniques are based on modern dance theories, modified by the principles of kinesiology.

This book is offered as a resource to all professionals who are dedicated to improving life during senescence.

EVA DESCA GARNET

Contents

Acknowledgments   vi
Foreword   viii
Introduction   xi

PART I: AGING AND MOBILITY

1   Gerontological Background   3
2   Health: One of the Joys of Life   6
3   Movement Throughout Life   10
4   The Paradox of Old Age: Inactivity vs. Health   15
5   Movement: Normal and Natural   18
6   Discovering the Senses Through Movement   28
7   Vitality or Senility?   36

PART II: THE GERIATRIC BODY DYNAMICS PROGRAM:
         PRINCIPLES AND METHODS

8   Geriatric Body Dynamics: A Movement Therapy   45
9   Teaching the Senescent Student   59
10   The Body as an Instrument   72
11   Communicating with Students   75
12   Improving Posture and Motor Skill   104
13   Guided Discussion   109
14   The Lecture Demonstration   115
15   Starting a Geriatric Body Dynamics Class   119
16   The Moment of Truth   141

Bibliography   145
Index   153

Introduction

THIS BOOK presents a therapeutic approach to movement for people over the age of sixty who are additionally influenced by physical limitations and/or mental attitudes which curtail their physical activity.

Its theory, method, and practice of teaching movement grow from a holistic view of the older person's geriatric problems and needs. It considers physical inactivity a prime cause of the boredom and atrophy characteristic of aging, and it considers motivation the chief need for maintaining the basic mobility so essential to self-dependence.

The method emphasizes physical and psychological security. It stimulates inactive men and women to move while they enjoy the safety and comfort of the seated position. Fear and pain dissolve from the stiffened areas of the body and rigid attitudes of the mind as freedom of movement increases during these chair exercises. The movement process is enriched by the use of biofeedback, guided imagery, and sensory-awareness techniques. These "holistic" experiences are replete with insights that improve the self-image.

Rediscovery of the pleasure of moving is the *short-term* goal. Enjoyment of movement grows into physical fitness and participation in sports and dance activities which older people can only enjoy when they already move with confidence. Such movement-readiness occurs when the older person feels reassured that he or she can move in safety and comfort. As each person's ability grows, he or she can decide whether to continue with the moderate exercises of our exercise program or to move on to other tempting activities.

The *long-term* goal of this method is the development of the kinesthetic sense, one way of restoring meaning to life and providing biologically essential activity at the same time. At the time of life when the acuity of all the other senses is diminishing, the exploration of the movement sense is revitalizing. In geriatric body dynamics classes, new awarenesses discovered through the kinesthetic sense can become a life-renewing, physically rejuvenating adventure.

PART I

Aging and Mobility

1
Gerontological Background

DURING the 1960s research in the universities and public agencies reflected an increased attempt to understand the biological nature of aging and the social nature of retirement. Biologists, sociologists, and psychologists developed a new language and new ideas around the young study of *gerontology,* the science dealing with aging and the special problems of older people.

The terms *biological aging* and *biological clock* changed the scientific measurement of human aging. Today people age not according to their number of birthdays, but according to their physical condition. The words *biological clock* suggest that a person is as old as his or her arteries, or spine, or any other organ system crucial to life. Put another way, people's "oldness" is determined not by how long they have lived, but by how soon they will die. A person of any age with advanced cardiovascular disease is older than a person of seventy who is free of this hazard.

Closely related to biological concepts of aging are the words *senescence* and *senility.* *Senescence* is the long life that everyone hopes for. It is part of the life cycle that lasts longer than infancy, childhood, and adolescence put together. *Senility,* on the other hand, represents a dreaded state of illness which is the most diseased aspect of age.

Retirement, the social condition that usually accompanies aging today, was widely debated throughout the 1960s. Gerontologists found that the happiness or unhappiness people experienced during retirement was determined not only by circumstances but also by beliefs and attitudes concerning the "work ethic."

Retirement, after all, means cessation of employment. Yet it does not bring to an end the belief that work is an expression of usefulness, meaningfulness, and status. The anthropologist, Margaret M. Clark (1968) wrote:

> Such values as youth, activity, multiple role involvement and independence, as well as productivity, are adverse to aging changes. Daily, we see the personal tragedies resulting from the contradiction between the contemporary needs of the elderly and these archaic attitudes towards a meaningful life.

The impossibility of viewing geriatric changes adaptively from these values is self-evident. These values are based upon the needs of youth and productivity, and they prepare people for their roles in the early part of the life cycle. They are not valid for the experience and behavior of people in the opposite end of the life cycle. It is not surprising that such conditions generate emotional conflict in older people. When the stresses of these conflicts become too great, they inevitably cause a mental breakdown.

The psychiatrist Dr. Alvin Goldfarb of Mt. Sinai Hospital (New York) developed a model of mental illness and senility as early as 1967. He charted the development of the social and personal aspects in the following schema.

TABLE I

COMPONENTS OF DISORDER: PSYCHODYNAMIC SEQUENCE

Loss of resources	Decreased capacity for mastery	Feelings of helplessness Fall in self-esteem and self-confidence	Fear Anger Fear of retaliation Guilt	Search for aid Dependency Parent substitute Regressive behavior

In an interview in 1970, Dr. Goldfarb explained this schema as follows:

> The feelings of helplessness are compounded by the damaged self-image due to the expectations he has learned to have of himself and others. . . .
> In answer to his question, "Who am I" he answers, "I am not what I should be, I have failed, I am ashamed, I feel guilty, I feel angry." The interaction of these feelings with those of grief at losses of persons and capacities occur as the older person becomes dependent.
> When the older person reacts with enough fear and anger he becomes a mental patient.

Thus we see that senility is not only a medical problem but also a social one. The loss of personal worth is related to the loss of social worth. Improvement in chances for health during senescence is largely dependent on changes in attitudes and opportunities for older people.

Social planners are attempting to remedy the situation. Programs based on new understanding of the aging process are increasingly attentive to the importance of the physical and emotional needs of older people. Efforts by creative professionals and service organizations are being funded by various government agencies to initiate constructive social attitudes and social opportunities for a meaningful lifestyle. Among these programs are: group dining at nutrition centers; a variety of relevant classes in "continuing education"; volunteer service jobs performed by older people; and group transportation for special trips and quality entertainment.

Significant attitudinal changes are occurring in still other arenas. Medicare funds going to convalescent homes are accompanied by "new regulations [requiring] . . . social and psychological care . . ." (Kramer and Kramer, 1976). The State of California has made compulsory retirement illegal. Television is presenting responsible coverage of rewarding new lifestyles.

These trends give older people an incentive to restructure their lives after retirement. They offer an opportunity to participate with their peers in meaningful ways that are validated by our society. Physical fitness is an integral part of this design for a more satisfying life in senescence.

2
Health: One of the Joys of Life

Health must be one of the joys of life
As no other joy is possible without it.
—THOMAS MORE, *Utopia*

THE SHANAS AND TOWNSEND study (1968) established that older people consider themselves healthy if they have two or less chronic diseases, can walk up and down stairs, care for their personal needs, and function independently with little or no pain. We refer to these people as the *well-aging*. Unfortunately, any illness can rob the older person of these essentials for independent living and catapult him or her into a hospital or nursing home where, after remaining under care for a while, the subject may join the *chronically ill*. In between these two groups is another identifiable subgroup: those who receive congregate care, such as people who live in retirement homes or board-and-care homes. Most of these people can be defined as well-aging but do not take full responsibility for independent living. They rely on the safety and services established in their residential contracts.

Health: One of the Joys of Life

Elderly people often face visual, auditory, physical, mental, or perceptual handicaps. Almost equally debilitating is the loss of adaptability to stress, which Hans Selye, father of the stress theory of illness, characterizes as the process of aging. While it is all too commonly assumed that sickness is the companion of old age, this is not necessarily so.

However, the fear of losing health and security can build a level of anxiety that paves the way for a whole train of somatic and psychological ills. Meaningful activity is believed to be the only antidote to premature aging and senility (Kleemeier, 1964). But for the millions of older people already handicapped, such activity must be tailored to accommodate their disabilities.

Movement therapy can help both the well-aging (in the open community) and the chronically ill (in their more sheltered situations). Professionals generally work with the well-aging in organized leisure-time activities. These may be sponsored by schools of adult education, parks and recreational commissions, senior citizen clubs, community centers, retirement homes, and other service organizations. Here, the participants attend the activity as long as it supplies them the sociability, variety, stimulation, recognition, and safety they seek.

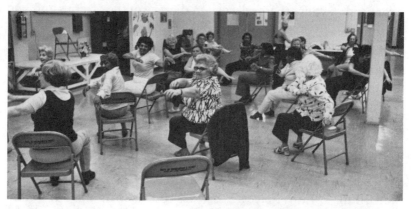

Figure 1. Members of a Senior Citizens' Club find stimulation and sociability in the Body Dynamics Class

The second group, who represent the physically and/or mentally impaired, are in nursing or convalescent homes or some other medically supervised facility. In such settings, one's physical space, or *life-space,* is a tiny world within the larger facility where normal activity comes nearly to a standstill. Most of these people have given up the world to seek relief from some form of constant distress. Here the goal of the professional is prevention of atrophy and senility.

Different as these two groups may be, the people in both have a common need for therapeutic supports. What function can movement therapy perform for both these groups? Before answering that question, we have to know something about the dynamics of *biological aging* (Birren, 1964). We need some information about normal movement patterns, the physical and psychological conditions, and practical scales to measure improvement. We should also have some reason for believing that movement therapy can improve the psychosomatic functioning of older people.

Biological aging, as we noted before, is equated with the functioning of the vital organ systems. The familiar expression, "You are as young as your arteries," implies that your age is as advanced as your atherosclerosis, a disease of the arteries and one of the causes of senility. Expressed organically, the closer a person's heart, lungs, or kidneys are to failure, the older he or she is biologically.

Stress and distress affect *homeostasis,* "the maintenance of a normal steady state in the body" (Selye, 1974). Chronic distress brings about adverse biological changes through the mechanism of prolonged *heterostasis, i.e.,* when one or more systems are responding to stress. Of course, disease causes distress as well as destruction, and the aging process becomes a vicious spiral. According to Hans Selye all distress results in aging, but not all stress is distressful. Some stress is essential and desirable. This he calls *eustress* (Selye, 1978).

Work is a biological necessity. Just as our muscles become flabby and degenerate, if not used, so our brain slips into chaos and confusion unless we constantly use it for work that seems worthwhile to us. . . .

Besides—as we have said earlier—certain types of activities have a curative effect and actually help to keep the stress mechanism in good shape.

It is well known that occupational therapy is one of the most efficient ways of dealing with certain mental diseases, and that exercise of your muscles keeps you fit. It all depends on the type of work you do and the way you react to it (Selye, 1975).

Selye differentiates work from labor by quoting George Bernard Shaw: "Labor is doing what we must; leisure is doing what we like." The meaning of work is in the doing, while the meaning of labor is in the earning. The physiological effect of enjoyable activity (eustress) affects heterostasis, the stress mechanism, favorably. It reverses the downward spiral and stimulates a beneficial chain reaction in the circulatory, respiratory, and nervous systems. After an enjoyable activity, the body at rest tends to return to homeostasis. Put simply, by improving the functioning of the participant's life-support systems, eustress retards biological aging.

People who are old are commonly expected to rest, and people who are both old and ill are expected to be bedridden. What happens when they are encouraged to move?

3
Movement Throughout Life

EVEN BEFORE the infant is born, we can feel it moving within the womb. Its first stirrings send a watchful mother into cries of delight. "I feel life!" she exclaims.

Then, after birth, before the infant can turn in his or her crib, little arms and legs swing and kick, reach and push; toes curl and fists clench. When, with pointed toes, the newborn child breaks into an unexpected whirlwind of pedaling, even a casual observer cannot resist the contagious joy of the sheer rhythmic outbursts. Untaught, the infant repeats these movements ritually, as though life itself depended on it.

Each baby demonstrates the biological importance of movement with every part of his or her incredibly active little body. Interacting with the world, the infant responds to a warm bath, cold sheets, a gentle caress, and an unexpected noise, with hands, feet, mouth, legs, spine, and every other movable part. The hungry child often adds a wail of frustration to the ever-growing repertory. But one blast never seems enough and is usually followed by a rhythmic variety of longs and shorts.

This rhythmic alarm is powered internally by a bellows of lungs, muscles, and nerves which is matched externally with lively contortions that mimic the internal contractions. The earliest response of the infant to comfort or discomfort, pleasure or pain, is expressed through an infinite combination of rhythmic movements.

Rhythm

Movement is essential to life, but is rhythm? In our culture, we associate the concept of rhythm with the arts. But art is dominated by nature, and the most vital sources of rhythm in art can be traced to our own rhythmic processes. The pulse and heartbeat influence tempo; inhalation and exhalation shape the phrase; chewing and swallowing give us staccato and legato; reproduction, from the long lunar rhythm of ovulation to the accelerated rhythms of conception, gives us our sense of climax. Also, how long can we go without moving our hands and feet— gesturing, shifting weight, walking with unconscious sureness?

Ordinarily all these automatic movements go unnoticed. Not until we experience a pounding heart, difficulty in breathing, or a spastic larynx do we become painfully aware of these processes. Perhaps this is why many older people associate movement awareness with pain.

Rhythmic movement is so essential to health and growth that it is built into our earliest behavior and grows as we do, through infancy, childhood, adolescence, adulthood, and senescence.

As infants, we master the skills of crawling, sitting, standing, walking, and running. Our insatiable curiosity drives us to manipulate things. And this curiosity is not satisfied until we have repeatedly dropped, thrown, opened, closed, squeezed, chewed, broken, and "fixed" everything at hand.

Then follow the better-remembered rhythmic experiences and feats of balance on teeter-totters, slides, skates, bikes, and in street games and sports. And so we move and act in an unending chain, increasing our coordination, strength, and balance well into maturity.

Our muscular strength grows from a combination of (1) power from what we do, and (2) energy from what we eat. Our need for food is instinctively reinforced by our appetite and assisted by the pleasure in tasting. Similarly, our biological need for movement is ensured by the sensation of pleasure in movement. Rhythm is a large part of that pleasure. Some say it is experienced before birth in the lub-dub of the mother's heartbeat. Whatever its root, rhythm is probably the most universally enjoyed characteristic of movement.

11

Play

In childhood, the need for movement is fulfilled by self-directed enjoyable activity. The child develops as he or she plays. The principle of self-directed, enjoyable movement understood as play is productive in every stage of life.

Many adults balance the tedious work for their livelihood with recreational activities they enjoy. These activities provide more than release from work. They establish interests essential for maintaining active lives after retirement. Others, who prefer to rest after work, develop habits that alienate them from movement.

The Law of Exercise

Injured or diseased children who can no longer move suffer a tragic wasting away of muscles. We have no difficulty recognizing the direct connection between the lack of use and the atrophy it causes in these young people, because the atrophy contrasts so strikingly with the natural process of growth.

Yet when we see the same wasting away in older people after injury or inactivity, we mistakenly assume this to be natural to old age. We miss the biological significance of periodic rhythmic exercise for older people.

It is well known that "use stimulates tissues to grow. Exercise causes greater development of muscle" (Stieglitz, 1962). "The more times the stimuli and responses are paired, the stronger is the association between the two" (Isaacson et al, 1965). Repetition is the key to physical learning and growth. The functional connection between the maintenance of muscle through use and the atrophy of muscle through disuse is the law of exercise.

Habit Versus Awareness

The fundamental motions of our daily lives are so intertwined with our habits that we are scarcely conscious of them. In this sense, our habits work for us. A skilled driver is concerned with safety in traffic, not the mechanical motions of shifting gears. The typist is concerned with communication, not the finger movements in hitting each key.

But the same trained movements can work against us. The abrupt change to retirement lops off an amazing amount of habitual activity. Even sedentary workers miss a whole repertory of comings and goings that are the woof and warp of the lifestyle of employment.

Upon retirement, what happens to the time previously filled with job-related activities? Often this free time is used for such sedentary pastimes as television, reading, resting, and sleeping. Meanwhile, just as people are unaware of the conditioning effect of their automatic work-a-day movements, they are equally unaware of the loss of these movements when they substitute sedentary activities for them.

Why are we not aware of our movements? First, because they become habitual, and second, we learn the basic motions of grasping, holding, sitting, and so on before we develop the psychological awareness of ourselves as individuals; that is, before we develop an ego. Since we do not remember learning these skills, we are unaware that we have to maintain them. For example, few of us have any idea of the number of motions we make every morning when we get out of bed. It might be fun to figure it out for yourself.

A Motion Study

Even if you are agile enough to stand on your feet by the count of three, you will have negotiated about twenty movements to get out of bed. If you happen to be lying on your back when you open your eyes, the sequence of movements might include the following:

1. bending the elbows to
2. reach the covers

3. flexing the wrists and fingers to
4. grasp the covers
5. lifting the shoulders in preparation for
6. throwing the covers back
7. extending the elbows, wrists, fingers in the act of
8. throwing the covers off
9. lifting the head up
10. twisting the spine toward the side to
11. roll over
12. helping to roll to the side by bending the knees and hips and
13. pushing with the feet to get to
14. sitting position at the edge of the bed
15. leaning forward
16. lifting the weight off the buttocks
17. to the feet
18. balancing on the feet
19. as the ankles, knees, hips, and spine extend the body upright
20. balancing to maintain this upright position

These movements describe only the action of the joints. There are at least three times as many muscles involved in negotiating these movements from the supine position in bed to the standing position on the floor.

One might ask that if automatic movements serve us so well, why should we become conscious of them? This simple motion study is of more than academic interest when discomfort or illness punctuate every bend of a joint or stretch of a muscle.

All of us have experienced painful sensations in moving at one time or another. But chronic pain experienced during movement is a familiar complaint of people who have *arthritis,* a disease of the joints. For many older people just getting out of bed is a painful ordeal.

Pain is a message that alerts us to a condition in need of correction. When movement is recommended as part of the therapy in treating people with arhtritis, the pain is often a deterrent to carrying out the instruction. Through geriatric body dynamics, teachers and therapists have an opportunity of helping people overcome the painful stiffness with a minimum of discomfort.

4

The Paradox of Old Age: Inactivity Versus Health

MOST OF the contradictions in a person's lifestyle seem to implode after retirement. For instance, although the time previously devoted to the job becomes free, many people do not experience this freedom as opportunity. Too often the unscheduled period remains empty time. With fewer demands and less activity, the tedium mounts, and daily life becomes sterile.

Movement becomes uncomfortable. Many older people give up the effort, feeling they deserve a rest. This results in the most fundamental paradox of aging. Instead of increasing the sense of well-being, inactivity gives rise to a sense of weakness. The rest, instead of refreshing, debilitates. As stiffness and pain prohibit freedom of movement, the body becomes a prison and rest becomes arrest.

In the life cycle, there is an increasingly emotional distance between the early ecstasy of movement and the later period when it can scarcely be endured. Yet the biological need for activity is ever present.

By the time older people understand the danger of this paradox, even if they are ready to join in recreational activities, they often find them too difficult or too strenuous. Before they can participate, the activities must be modified to their abilities and needs by therapists. What they once enjoyed as *recreation* is now *therapy*.

Paradoxically, one may spend a lifetime of striving for comfort in old age, only to discover that it is such simple activities as getting out of bed, striding forward, climbing stairs, and entering a car that become the most valued assets in surviving with comfort and pleasure.

In youth, pain is recognized as a signal. It is a cue to rest the injured part so as to promote the healing process. So, as we get older, we heed the signal and begin to rest all the parts that hurt. Instead of relieving pain, however, the inactivity only heightens discomfort. According to Dr. Roman L. Yanda, Rehabilitation Director of the Sherman Oaks Hospital (California), in later life the automatic response of rest to pain is maladaptive. Most aching muscles and joints get worse if they are not moved.

In time pain and weakened muscles from inactivity cause a *postural set* characterized by the contracture of the unused muscles, and ligaments that connect the boney frame of the body. The sagging upper back results in the aged look that a child once described as "bent over little." In this postural set, an elderly person stands with his or her feet widely separated to increase the base for better balance. The hips are thrust to the back. This results in an angle at the hips that deprives leg movements of the power of the buttocks during walking. The wide base results in a waddle that denies the hips and lower back of the benefits of rhythmic torque or twist.

The steps of such an older person are small, because of the fear of falling. Eyes are focused on the ground for the same reason. This affects the equilibrium and makes the balance less steady, because the floor seems to be moving as the feet progress forward.

Anxiety, caused by fear of falling or pain, inhibits all

movement, including breathing. People usually hold their breath during movements that require increased effort or concentration. This can result in improper breathing while moving up or down stairs, looking for a misplaced object, or learning something new. Breath-holding adds distress to the original effort.

Similarly harmful are the acts of looking and listening which are not aided by a pattern of neck and spine-twisting movements. Without this mobility the instant panoramic field of peripheral sights and sounds is lost. Instead, a slower, laborious movement of the body-as-a-whole turns to respond. "Many older people have accidents on stairs and in bathrooms owing to changes in eye-muscle teamwork. The muscles are slower to respond; the eyes misjudge near distances" (Lawton, 1956).

This slower movement pattern deprives the neck and torso of the torque that maintains the flexibility of the upper spine. The loss of movement, in turn, reduces circulation in the area. At the same time, older people also tend to restrict their elbow movements. Most arm gestures avoid the sidewise lift of the elbow (abduction) because of social restraints. Eating, drinking, reaching up with the hands are increasingly accomplished by bending the elbows in front of the body. This hikes up the shoulders, thereby using the much abused trapezius and levator scapulae muscles at the back and neck instead of using the appropriate deltoid, teres, and rhomboid muscles which strengthen the upper arm and upper back. Except for a few overused muscles in the neck and shoulder, the muscles and joints of the upper torso are neglected and contribute to the "bent over little" effect.

The backward rotation of the pelvis deprives the organs of the abdomen of pelvic support, and they rely only on abdominal muscles. This constant weight and pressure of the viscera forces the abdominal muscles to stretch. The organs sag as the abdominal muscles weaken. The lower back, which needs the support of strong abdominal muscles, weakens as well.

All the above habits combine to establish the postural set associated with old age. In turn, the postural set is the mold that shapes all the other movements the person normally makes. It should be clear from the normal movement patterns already described that the movement repertory of most older people is not serving even the minimum requirement for efficient biological function or physical safety.

As therapists, we pursue a process of change from normal patterns of movement that are maladaptive and wasteful to more natural movement patterns that promote healthy body function and are life-supporting.

5

Movement: Normal and Natural

NORMAL REFERS to a behavior characteristic of a large population. *Normal* is that which is predictable because the expectations are socially and educationally conditioned. The meaning of *normal* also extends to an act of one individual. In repeating an act many, many times, the act becomes predictable as a habit.

Natural, on the other hand, refers to a behavior characteristic of the homeostatic needs. *Natural* relates to biologically determined expectations. This meaning extends to any act that promotes the proper functioning of the body, which we call *health.*

To these definitions we must add other implied meanings.

Many people believe that if something is normal it must be right, because most people are doing it. And if it is natural, it must be good, because nature is God's work. People often use the two words interchangeably. It follows then that a person who believes his or her activity is normal thinks it is both good and right.

During the first months of life the natural is normal when an infant is breast-fed on demand. As we age, however, we adapt to society. Our natural impulses are inhibited as "normal behavior" predominates.

Though the two words continue to be used synonymously, they increasingly describe opposite effects. The harmful results of this confusion can be seen in the following illustration.

At the age of 72, Berdie, a mother and widow, retired from her small business in which she had taken care of her business records, banking, ordering, stocking, and selling. She had also been an active homemaker, as well as politically and socially involved.

Now, several years later, she lives alone and takes care of her three-room apartment, where she prepares her own meals, entertains her friends, and belongs to a health club. When friends ask what she does all day, she answers guiltily, "I don't know. Nothing, I guess." In comparing her present activity to her busy life before retirement, she underestimates it. But in terms of essential activity even the first 10 minutes of a visit with Berdie are revealing.

Breakfast Preparation: Motion-Time Study

Berdie greets me at the door, invites me to join her for breakfast, and heads for the kitchen to get it started. The room is about nine steps long by three steps wide, so she does quite a bit of walking just going back and forth from the sink at one end to the oven at the other.

Figure 2. Diagram of Berdie's kitchen.

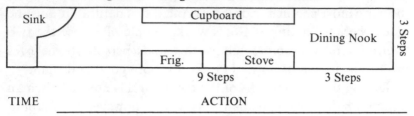

TIME	ACTION
9:00	Walk into kitchen, take coffee pot, carry to gas range. Twist gas jet. Bend over to see if flame is on. Walk to closet. Bend over, look for fry pan on bottom shelf. In this postition about 20 seconds. Walk to stove with fry pan.
9:05	Walk to refrigerator. Bend over to look for bacon and eggs. Open package of bacon. Separate slices. To lay the slices on pan, use fingers, arms, and eyes, and change weight from side to side. Turn gas jet, adjust flame.
9:10	Stretch arms to reach above back burner. Place pan with bacon on flame. Walk to closet. Get bread. Use saw knife to cut bread. Move arms from shoulder.
9:15	Bend to put bread into oven to toast. Get napkins and silverware, bring to table in dining nook.

She continues 15 more minutes of talking, fetching, carrying, opening, closing, lifting and lowering, twisting, beating, looking for and finding, matching and arranging. As she serves the steaming breakfast of bacon and eggs, buttered toast, hot chocolate, and prunes, she urges me to eat it while it's hot.

While we cannot measure the quality of pleasure and pride that occurred in this activity, we can record and quantify the basic movements. It is amazing how much stretching, contracting, stabilizing, and holding is involved in these movements. They maintain the flexibility and strength in the muscles and contribute to the beneficial effect that 30 minutes of standing and walking has on the maintenance of bone strength.

The following results record and tally six movements of the many diverse patterns Berdie performed.

TABLE II
TABULATION OF SIX BASIC MOVEMENTS
DURING MOTION-TIME STUDY

Movement:	Walking steps	Lift and carry	Bend	Push and pull	Reach	Turn
Number of Times:	149	61	14	25	12	37

While we were eating, I entertained Berdie by reading the description of her movements. She was very interested and commented on how much a person does automatically without being aware of it.

Within a short time Berdie gave up her apartment to move into a board and care home. Most of her time was spent sitting— sitting and reading, sitting and eating, sitting and watching television, sitting in the patio, sitting and visiting.

The biggest upsurge of activity was the morning grooming, walking to and from meals, and walking to and from the bathroom. But everyone else was doing the same thing, so Berdie's inactivity was "normal."

Notice how the concept of *normal* is group-dominated. Before retirement, an active life was normal. After retirement, an adequately active life did not seem normal. In Berdie's new "home," an inactive life was normal. Yet none of these "normal" conditions have supported her natural needs properly. They are neither good nor right.

This study describes the movement patterns performed habitually in the active retirement of the homemaker. It gives us some idea of the time and activity required for a single chore, that of preparing breakfast. It demonstrates the kind of muscular movement involved, and the extent of movement performed. It implies the amount of activity that is lost when such minimal tasks are excluded from her lifestyle. And, most importantly, it quantifies the amount of bending, stretching, twisting, weight changing, and locomotion that has to be built into an exercise program to supplement the inactive lifestyle.

As therapists, we can help the great majority of well-aging people. We can free the older person who is sandwiched in the normal/natural fallacy so that he or she can realistically pursue a healthier, appropriately active course. We can urge growing support for the *therapeutic community* which creates a new norm of activity consistent with functional health restoration and maintenance for the chronically ill population.

In working with the geriatric population, we emphasize physical action that helps regulate the life processes of the body. In Figure 3a the bodily processes benefited by movement are in one circle called *Life Processes*. The basic movement patterns of the body are in another circle called *Physical Movement*. In Figure 3b both circles intersect to form an interface. This area represents the regulatory benefits of movement to the life processes.

To illustrate the cardiovascular effect of movement, let us consider a biofeedback exercise for a well-aging class. Using a stopwatch to monitor the procedure, the students are instructed to feel the tiny pulsating movements at the wrist or throat and to count their own "resting pulse" (Morehouse and Gross, 1976). The participants prepare for the exercise by moving forward to the front edge of the seat. They are then asked to stand up and sit down repeatedly for one minute.

Each combination takes four seconds: two to stand, two to sit. Breathe in to stand; breathe out to sit. The combined breathing and stand/sit exercise is performed fifteen times in the minute. At the end of this period, most of the members of the class have increased their "action pulse rate" by ten to thirty beats per minute over their "resting pulse rate." This exercise increases

Physical Movement

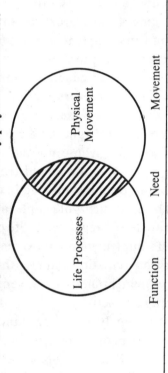

bending—extending
contracting—releasing
pulling—pushing
twisting—turning
falling—bouncing
swinging—swaying
expanding—squeezing
rocking—weight change
touching—holding
tapping—sliding
standing—walking
jumping—running
hopping—stamping
letting go

Life Processes

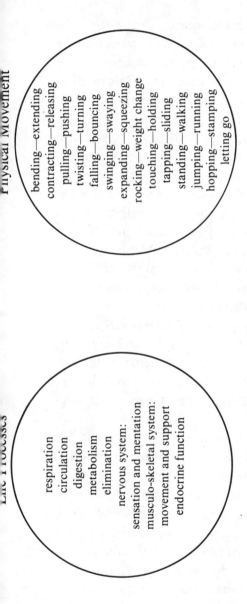

respiration
circulation
digestion
metabolism
elimination
nervous system:
sensation and mentation
musculo-skeletal system:
movement and support
endocrine function

Figure 3a Life processes benefited by physical movement

Life Processes

Physical Movement

Function   Need   Movement

Figure 3b. Interface between life processes and physical movement

cardiovascular activity and benefits both the breathing and musculoskeletal systems.

The improvements in circulation, deeper breathing, the "milking action" of the thigh muscles on the veins, as well as the other benefits to the muscles and joints, are talked about in the discussion period following the exercise. This information increases interest and appreciation of body movement and body messages and acts as a further incentive to exercise.

Figure 4 conceptualizes the way the two basic lifestyles in aging—independent retirement and dependent retirement—relate to and promote organic function. The left-hand circle represents the well-aging population whose normal activities of grooming, chores, recreation, service to others, walking, social activities, trips, exercise, and sex help regulate their bodily processes. The right-hand circle represents the older people who require care, whose normal activity has shrunk to ablutions, grooming, walking to and from meals, standing up and sitting down, or even just moving in a wheelchair.

The movements of people in the latter group are insufficient to stimulate and regulate the life processes. These dependent people need supplementary movement exercises particularly for improved circulation and breathing. For them, and those who live in retirement homes, movement supplement becomes a life-supporting activity.

Fortunately, changing standards of normal physical behavior for older people are evolving along with a holistic view of the problem. Professionals are establishing activities for people in communities, in retirement homes, and particularly in convalescent hospitals that meet requirements for increased physical, psychological, and emotional stimulation at the same time.

The most advanced convalescent hospitals have initiated the holistic concept of the *therapeutic community* (Kramer and Kramer, 1976). This approach to long-term care requires special teamwork involving changes in attitude and behavior of all the

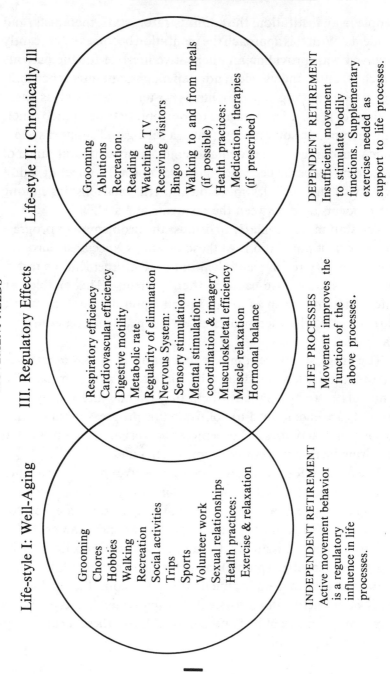

Movement: Normal and Natural

DAILY NORMAL MOVEMENT
BEHAVIOR AND NATURAL
MOVEMENT NEEDS

Life-style I: Well-Aging

Grooming
Chores
Hobbies
Walking
Recreation
Social activities
Trips
Sports
Volunteer work
Sexual relationships
Health practices:
Exercise & relaxation

INDEPENDENT RETIREMENT
Active movement behavior
is a regulatory
influence in life
processes.

III. Regulatory Effects

Respiratory efficiency
Cardiovascular efficiency
Digestive motility
Metabolic rate
Regularity of elimination
Nervous System:
Sensory stimulation
Mental stimulation:
coordination & imagery
Musculoskeletal efficiency
Muscle relaxation
Hormonal balance

LIFE PROCESSES
Movement improves the
function of the
above processes.

Life-style II: Chronically Ill

Grooming
Ablutions
Recreation:
Reading
Watching TV
Receiving visitors
Bingo
Walking to and from meals
(if possible)
Health practices:
Medication, therapies
(if prescribed)

DEPENDENT RETIREMENT
Insufficient movement
to stimulate bodily
functions. Supplementary
exercise needed as
support to life processes.

Figure 4. Model of movement as a life-support

25

people in an institution: the administrator, staff, therapists, and residents. With this approach the institution becomes significantly involved with providing an alternative lifestyle for the patients which is neither independent nor dependent, but interdependent. Interaction among the patients is fostered which gives them options of greater freedom and responsibility toward each other. The therapeutic community creates a caring and support system which encourages its residents to enjoy a more natural range of emotional experiences and a more normal range of adult activities. This includes more meaningful relationships among the residents, and between the residents and staff.

The staff meets regularly to discuss the problems and progress of the patient population. At these meetings, specialists have the opportunity to recommend the kind of reinforcement the rest of the staff should give each of their patients. This enables an integration of influences on the hospital population. It permits a carry-over of the therapeutic effect of the group sessions into daily life.

The progress a patient makes in a group session is recognized by the nurses, nurse's aides, administrators, and everyone else who relates to the patient, including friends and family. The patients are encouraged to continue this progress in their other groups and activities. They enjoy the verbal recognition that confirms their own feelings of improvement.

The positive feedback that each one receives becomes part of a healing process. In a therapeutic community each person has a therapeutic effect on the other and helps "the older person (patient) live fully until he dies . . ." (Kramer and Kramer, 1976).

This, of course, is an ideal situation. At the opposite pole are the convalescent hospitals that offer their patients little more than custodial care under medical supervision. This includes a daily bath, medication, physical therapy (when prescribed by a physician), change of bed and personal linen, three meals a day, television, visits from family and friends, bingo, and attention to some requests and complaints.

A good therapist evaluates the facility's concern and service to its patients and emphasizes those aspects of movement therapy that gratify the most prevalent needs. Patients in some facilities may feel especially lonely and may need greater interaction with others through movement. Disengagement,i.e., a loss of interest in environment and other people, may be a predominant symptom. Sensory stimulation through movement, sounds, and touch is more productive with these patients. In still other facilities opportunities to relieve pent-up feelings through vigorous movement get the best response.

The foregoing suggestions concern emphasis not exclusiveness. Interaction, sensory stimulation, and catharsis are therapeutically significant for all groups.

One word about normalcy in convalescent hospitals: many wheelchair patients have catheters attached to urinal bags that are suspended on the chair. Many of these patients display as much movement potential as other wheelchair patients. They are lucid and very enthusiastic about the mental stimulation they experience along with the excitement of the exercise.

6
Discovering the Senses Through Movement

Mind and Body

GRANTED that exercise is essential to maintain a sound body, but what has movement to do with the mind?

"I think; therefore I am," said the French philosopher, Descartes. With this statement he established the concept of the independence from, and superiority of, the mind over the body. This separation dominated scientific thought for 250 years.

William James, father of classical American psychology, challenged this view by presenting his own observations about the unity of the mind and body.

All mental states ... are followed by bodily activity of some sort. They lead to inconspicuous changes in breathing, circulation, general muscular tension, and glandular and other visceral activity ... even mere thoughts and feelings are motor in their consequences.

We can easily recognize the motor effects of emotion. All of us walk faster when we are eager to get someplace. We move with increased strength when we are determined. When we are frightened, we hold our breath, become rigid, or pull into a smaller shape to become less conspicuous. When we are happy, we bounce along effortlessly.

Sense Through Movement

Our psychological behavior is accompanied by or expressed through movement. The will to see, hear, taste, smell, touch, and, of course, move, involves a series of head, axial (torso), and pendular (arms or legs) movements.

For instance, the eye muscles involved in looking are generally accompanied by an ensemble of neck muscles. These muscles shorten or lengthen to permit vision of the sky, ground, or objects in between and all around. Our own head, torso, or legs take us closer to or farther away from the sounds and smells we like or dislike. Similarly, the potential to taste food and touch surfaces can only be achieved through movement.

While the movement or *kinesthetic* sense, like the other senses, is perceived in the brain, it differs in several ways from the other senses. An interesting difference is the kind of information it relays.

The other five senses are *exteroceptors,* informing the mind of the external environment. They are in contact with the outside, and their organs are found in observable parts of the body: the eyes, nose, ears, mouth, and skin.

The movement sense reveals information of the internal environment through the components of movement, the nerves and muscles which are threaded throughout the body making the whole body the sense organ of movement. This implies that the movement sense, through the body-as-a-whole, underlies the other sense organs; and that we experience them through movement.

Our awareness of movement in relation to the other senses enables us to focus on the smallest voluntary movement experiences of seeing, smelling, swallowing, touching, and breathing. Once we gain the skill to sense these, it becomes comparatively easy to separate out the specific movement experiences of weight, pressure, force, direction, space, timing, and relaxation.

Movement in a direction becomes an experience in spatial relationships. As we lean, bend, stretch, or move into space, we get a sense of near and far, here and there, in relation to our bodies and body parts. Our timing develops with our sense memory. We can differentiate the memory of fast from slow as we move, and even from uneven as we walk. We experience duration, or long and short, as we breathe. And the exhalation which permits speech governs the length of the spoken phrase.

The sensation of pressure and weight enables us to feel the ground, to be aware of the contact. We perceive it as a firm base of support by relaxing into it or pushing against it. This interaction or bonding with the ground is called *grounding*. It facilitates a muscle sense of balance which, together with vestibular (ears) and visual (eyes) input, form the sense of equilibrium. This physical experience of balance is fundamental to another basic mind/body sensation, *centering*. *Centering* is the awareness of a drawing toward center, with the center the point around which anything revolves or pivots. In the torso, the pivotal points are along its core, the spinal column. Centering represents a sense of balance through the spine at rest or in action.

Centering and grounding are both psychologically significant when they become tools adapted to cope with conflicts and problem solving. They are a physical process for regaining a sense of stability and reality which is often threatened by such stressful situations. These two principles are part of the philosophy of Gestalt therapy. "...Healthy living is a process of creative adjustment. To be able to be grounded in this process and live with it is maturity ... to be centered is to deal with the circumstances of our lives ... according to the dictates of healthy functioning ..." (Latner, 1972).

Our movement sense communicates through three feelings— *push, pull,* and *let go*—and through the active and passive combinations that result from them. When we move and continue to observe our own behavior, we may discover that we characteristically enjoy pushing or pulling, or that we enjoy being pushed or pulled. The ability to let go, with which we have varying degrees of success, makes possible such other movements as swinging, bouncing, suspension, and momentum—the exhilarating movements.

If we are guided to focus on sensing through movement, we may become aware that these feelings flow over into our relations with others. These simple movements can help us to understand our personalities. Do we like to push or be pushed? Do we like to pull or be pulled? Do we prefer to let go and permit events to happen to us?

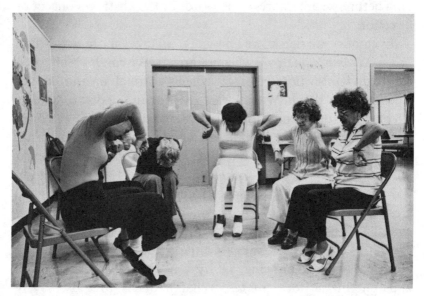

Figure 5. Enjoying a dynamic experience of pushing and pulling in safety

How do we make sense from our movement? Concentrating on the twenty-six muscles of facial expression, we become aware that not only do our faces broadcast our feelings but we can read many clear messages in the smiling, pouting, or scowling expressions of other people's faces. This is equally true of the rest of the expressive movements of the body. If we accept William James' principle that motion precedes emotion, then each one of us is an open book to be understood through the meanings of our most subtle movements. The idea of body language is becoming accepted today, but it takes body-awareness to sense the meaning of its silent vocabulary.

Turning again to verbal communication, we know our language is studded with imagery, the meanings of which are derived from the body and its movement experiences. We experience the feeling of up and down, forward and backward, long before we are aware of the words or the abstract concept of direction.

From our experience, we know that *up* takes more effort than *down*. We can look down when we are up. We can look up when we are down. We become bigger when we stretch up and smaller when we bend down. We can leap up. We can fall down. It takes effort to leap up but no effort to let go and fall down. We can drop into a chair and relax or fall and hurt ourselves. The internal information we experience through moving gives meaning to phrases such as up and down, high and low, look up to, look down on, leaping ahead, dropping back, aspire to greater heights, crestfallen, hold your head high, down in the mouth, and countless other expressions.

But our internal meanings are enlarged with the sophisticated meanings added to our language by our culture. This is especially apparent in the idea, *to fall.* What happens to those lovely meanings of letting go that we sense in "to fall asleep," "to fall in love?" We see the ease of letting go, relaxing, and falling disappear as negative meanings attach themselves to the idea, such as dropped, fell on his face, fallen woman, fallen hero, fall guy, dropped his head in shame, groveled on the floor, fell to his knees, lowering oneself.

All these negative images, emphasizing disdain or fear of falling, have a devastating influence on one-third of our movement sense, that of letting go and relaxing. *Letting go*

32

becomes undesirable behavior, and the price we pay for this senseless judgement ranges from discomfort to major psychosomatic diseases.

Part of the correction of this faulty judgment depends on our ability to "listen" to our body and interpret its messages. As we increase our body-awareness through movement, we cultivate an instrument capable of "hearing" inner cues of tension and stress. We can choose to redirect our energy to reduce the stress, or we can respond to the need to relax.

This is the basis of the holistic concept of health. It is founded on three premises: (1) the belief that the mind and body are mirrors of each other; (2) the capacity to change the behavior of one by changing the behavior of the other; (3) the assumption that the body has genetic information to maintain or regain its health, and the wisdom to communicate changes in its state of health through body signals of distress or pleasure.

If we value our internal messages, we can sense the feelings that pull us in one direction or push us in another. We can redirect our energy to *ground* and *center* ourselves during the creative effort essential for adapting to changing circumstances. And we can trust those choices that coincide with a feeling of centeredness.

Another way we make meaning from the kinesthetic sense is through the social attribute, *empathy.* This is the ability to sense the bodily feelings of others through the memory and identification of similar feelings in ourselves. Such experiences deepen our relationship with people. Empathy also intensifies our ability to respond to the movement of others.

Just as music appreciation is the reward of more discriminating hearing, movement appreciation is the reward of developed kinesthetic feeling. The enjoyment of movement skills in the arts and sports depends on this capacity to empathize. It increases our satisfaction whether we participate in the activities or merely watch.

The Holistic Concept of Mind and Body

The unifying view of mind and body, known as "a holistic model of health care," is a means of harnessing the body-as-a-whole for the prevention of disease and the promotion of recovery. "Several major medical researchers of this century, such as Claude Bernard, Harold G. Wolff, Ivan Pavlov, Walter B. Cannon, Hans Selye, and A.T.W. Simeons, have created a substantial foundation for a more compehensive understanding of the relationship between body and mind" (Pelletier, 1977).

For example, the contrasting emotions of anger and fear are part of the fight-or-flight response, "one of the body's most sensitive and vital survival systems" (Pelletier, 1977). These reactions cause predictable physiological effects. In fear, the adrenal glands release adrenaline "(which) dilates the arterials of the heart and skeletal muscles, and accelerates the heart rate . . ." The opposite reaction occurs when anger releases noradrenaline which "normally constricts the arterials and raises the blood pressure" (Pelletier, 1977).

This point of view maintains that susceptibility to disease is stress-related. And conversely, that body-awareness (the ability to read body messages) and intelligent stress-management (the avoidance of prolonged anger and fear responses) are the first lines of defense against disease. Body wisdom and stress-management are the psychological cornerstones of holistic preventive medicine.

The holistic movement emphasizes the power each person has in maintaining and improving his or her own health. For example, a person with high blood pressure who learns to react flexibly to a provoking situation can avoid the dangerous increase in blood pressure which is triggered by anger. It is becoming clear that the *mental-set,* how a person is poised to react to a given situation, i.e., fear, anger, or confidence, determines whether a positive result of wellness or a negative result of illness will occur.

The growing public interest in this view of health was proven in 1975 by the first national conference on holistic health care sponsored by the Rockefeller Foundation. The main question discussed was, "How can people achieve a level of well-being that will prevent the most serious and costly diseases....Leading health professionals including physicians, government officials, and insurance company executives ... (answered). Individuals must begin assuming responsibility for their own health and learning ways to maximize vitality and longevity. The whole person including physical, emotional, and spiritual dimensions must be considered" (Bloomfield, 1978).

The basic assumption of the holistic approach is the recognition of the two-way traffic of equal influence between the body and mind. When this approach is a guide to developing a sense of well-being it is called holistic health; when it is the guide in diagnosing and treating illness it is called holistic medicine.

The mental involvement in psychomotor activity, which influences the central nervous system at all ages (Hebb, 1966), makes muscular innervation and body-awareness exercises especially important in senescence. It exemplifies the principle of *Gestalt Psychology* that the whole is more than the sum of its parts. An exercise that involves conscious thought continues to benefit the parts of the body that are physically active, while it vitalizes the whole person, i.e., the mental, emotional, and spiritual dimensions of that person as a social human being.

7
Vitality or Senility?

SENESCENCE and the feeling of vitality need not be contradictory. This combination is not only possible, but it is the goal of successful aging. According to Dr. George Lawton, older people can be self-motivated or aided to continue to be active and grow in their ideas and relationships (Lawton, 1956).

Let us look at the spectrum of feelings diagrammed, for simplicity, as a psychosomatic continuum. The schematic presentation of this continuum in senescence (Figure 6) provides a practical scale for visualizing therapeutic improvement. The continuum is expressed as a straight line divided in half. The halfway point is marked zero. This is labeled *homeostasis,* the steady state. To the left of zero, the feeling of ill-functioning increases up to 100 percent, which is designated *senility.* To the right, the feeling of well-being increases up to 100 percent, termed *vitality.*

At zero, the state of homeostasis indicates that at rest all the systems of the body are functioning properly and are interacting harmoniously. To the left of zero, the continuous state of *distress* indicates that one or more systems is not functioning properly and cannot recover from a stressor. Homeostasis is disrupted. As the ill-functioning increases, *chronic illness* leads to *anxiety,* which may deepen to *depression.* If the depression goes unrelieved, it can finally result in complete dependence and *senility.*

The well-functioning side of the continuum starts at *eustress,* a state of beneficial stimulation during activity. *Health* indicates proper functioning during activity and return to homeostasis during rest. Proper stimulation increases a sense of *well-being,* and is maintained through physical and emotional *balance.* At this point, people can feel *exhilaration* through more intense

Vitality or Senility?

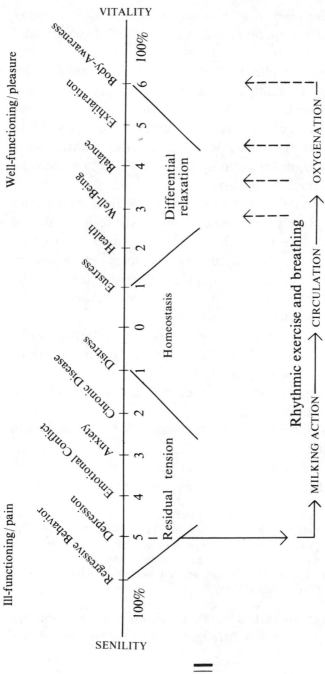

Figure 6. Psychosomatic continuum in senescence: a schematic presentation

experiences. The *body-awareness* required for the skill or ability to achieve such experiences is experienced physically and emotionally as *vitality*.

The continuum implies that continuing changes are possible from one point to another along the line. A well-functioning person may move between the steady state of homeostasis and the stimulated state of exhilaration. Such a fortunate person is in a steady state during sleep and wakes up refreshed with a sense of well-being. He or she feels healthy most of the time, and recovers quickly from temporary illness.

In eustress, the well-functioning person quickly regains a sense of balance physically and mentally. He or she feels capable of coping with daily events. The energy not wasted in needless tension or repairs due to distress is spent in rewarding experiences. The feeling of coping with responsibilities mentally and physically, at a time when many of one's peers are not, gives one additional feelings of self-validation.

All things being equal, we may assume that the healthy person's movements are generally free of pain, and that he or she seeks and enjoys fulfilling experiences.

Any of these states, even if temporary, may be considered a condition of optimal functioning.

The ill-functioning side of the continuum, starting with distress, implies certain physiological changes. The hormonal deficiency caused by the menopause or climacteric coincides with a great many discomforts and the loss of bone strength in women.

The commonest forms of osteoporosis in the elderly is the post-climacteric form ... It is believed that the condition is due to a lack of stimulation of the osteoblasts owing to deficiency of estrogen. Women are affected four times as frequently as men. This is presumably related to the earlier occurrence of the natural climacteric in women ... "Disuse atrophy" is another factor responsible for osteoporosis (Exton-Smith, 1955).

Recent research by Aiken et al, confirming the relationship between estrogen and bone strength, is reported in *The Clinical*

Management of Osteoporosis (Gordon and Vaughan, 1976).

The onset of the climacteric also has social implications. Among many men and women it means a poorer self-image, and a loss of self-esteem because of culturally molded attitudes toward virility and femininity. According to Dr. Alex Comfort, there are a "whole battery of unconscious fears among the non-old that are internalized by the older people and then turned against themselves." These attitudes and changes intensify feelings of anxiety and tension which, in turn, aggravate chronic illness (Comfort, 1970).

Unrelieved emotional conflict, anxiety, and resentment lead, according to Dr. Alvin Goldfarb, to depression. Then, especially during senescence, the subject may move from depression to regressive behavior to senility. This completes the downward spiral of ill-functioning in the psychosomatic continuum.

Experiences of improvement are subjective, often gleaned from the spontaneous comments of the participants in a geriatric body dynamics class, such as: "I feel a tingling sensation" (improved circulation); "I feel warm" (improved oxygen exchange); "I feel relaxed" (release of tension); "I feel exhilarated" (all of the foregoing, plus pleasure). When such comments are not spontaneous, the leader can question the participants directly.

In medically supervised facilities this information, along with other observations such as "decrease in complaints" or "less need for assistance," can be charted for each individual along with other reported objective measurements. Continuing improvement over an extended period increases the participants' self-esteem and ego-strength, even in patients still suffering from chronic disease and varying degrees of dependency.

Aging is a developmental process (Erikson, 1963). Every person fortunate enough to live a long life will eventually reach the senescent state. Consequently, all the handicaps and diseases to which people are heir are represented among the aged with whom we work. This includes all the categorical handicaps: the blind, deaf, mentally retarded, and so forth. But the diseases that head the list are cardiovascular: atherosclerosis or arteriosclerosis, hypertension, stroke, and heart attacks. These are followed by arthritis, diabetes, osteoporosis, Parkinson's disease, cancer, and various mental states including depression.

Disorientation and hallucination, considered mental symptoms of senility, may be symptoms of drug use and/or sensory deprivation, as recent research has shown. A collection of laboratory experiments are reported in the book *Sensory Deprivation: Fifteen Years of Research*. Following are some excerpts which substantiate the relevance of sensory deprivation to abnormal mental behavior:

> Murphy, Meyers and Smith of the Human Resources Research Office report that the young healthy men chosen as "subjects for the studies were soldiers at Fort Ord ... Subjects were isolated for a period of 96 hours in dark sound-proof cubicles and tested at various periods ... a significant number reported hallucinations."
>
> In "experimental reports describing effects of sensory deprivation ... originating at McGill University (Canada) ... subjects had complicating hallucinations and showed intellectual and perceptual deterioration" (Zubek, 1969).
>
> Sensory deprivation by immersion in water tanks, studies pioneered by John C. Lilly in 1956, reported profound effects including hallucination ... (Zubek, 1969).

Woodburn Heron, in *Scientific American,* reports:

> Experiments of sensory deprivation including sight, hearing, touch and movement on college male students reveal:
>
> After several days of isolation the whole room appeared to be in motion.
>
> The individual's thinking is impaired; he shows childish emotional responses; his visual perception becomes disturbed; he suffers from hallucinations; his brain wave pattern changes. These findings are in line with recent studies of the brain, especially of the reticular

formation of the mid-brain. (See "Pleasure Centers in the Brain" by James Olds, "Scientific American," Oct. 1956.) The recent studies indicate that normal functioning of the brain depends on a continued arousal reaction generated in the reticular formation which in turn depends on constant sensory bombardment."

It appears that aside from their specific functions, sensory stimuli have the general function of maintaining this arousal, and they rapidly lose their power to do so if they are restricted to the monotonously repeated stimulation of an unchanging environment. Under these circumstances . . . the brain behaves abnormally (Heron, 1957).

In older people, increasing blindness and deafness, loss of taste buds, the decrease of the tactile sensations associated with affectionate relationships, and loss of kinesthetic sensations from lack of activity all add up to massive sensory deprivation. Although we cannot restore lost senses, we can stimulate those that still function to help keep contact with reality.

Significant relationships, important throughout life, are even more important to older people. Most men and women sixty-five and over function quite well, as long as they enjoy rewarding experiences with relatives and friends. But companionship is not forever. Yesterday's wife is today's widow. Last year's celebration is replaced by this year's greeting card. Each year produces its own crop of losses.

Group experience can counteract the depressing effects of such social deprivation. People can help people. The group process that promotes interaction and meaningful relationships restores interest and excites anticipation. When these emotions are stimulated during movement classes, temporary transformations from depression to exhilaration become regular occurrences. Over a period of time, this practice generates a feeling of vitality.

PART II

The Geriatric Body Dynamics Program: Principles and Methods

8
Geriatric Body Dynamics: A Movement Therapy

COUNTERACTING the popular notion that old people hate to exercise, Geriatric Body Dynamics (GBD) has pioneered in creating an image of exercise that is attractive. GBD is a ritualized experience of rhythmic movement designed to overcome resistance by making the exercise experience practical, enjoyable, and therapeutically effective. Leaders of this program come from many disciplines and are variously referred to in this text as therapists, teachers, facilitators, or leaders. Its teaching methods and movement techniques are adapted to the biological, psychological, and sociological needs and limitations of older people—particularly their physical tolerance of stress and psychological need for support, contact, and good humor.

Psychological Techniques

GBD starts from five premises:

1. Everybody needs to exercise, but older people need to exercise in groups.
2. During every stage of life from infancy to old age, each person has characteristic needs. Our aim is for participants to experience exercise as relevant to their needs during senescence.
3. Older people who need supplementary movement the most are those least inclined to participate. As a result, movement specialists must be concerned with the psychological aspects of motivation.
4. The geriatric population needs therapeutic support for a variety of individual psychosomatic problems. But as a

group they also share similar physical and psychological needs:

a. Improvement of physical condition
b. Reduction of tension and anxiety
c. Increase of physical contact
d. Reduction of feelings of isolation and boredom
e. Conservation of adaptive energy

5. By specific movements involving physical contact with self, in partners, and in a group, participants can interact and have a therapeutic effect on each other.

Six Principles

Given these five premises, we can establish six basic principles for GBD. We term these principles "the six s's": *supplement, stimulation, safety, support, significance,* and *satisfaction.* For instance, retired people who experience a critical decrease in bodily activity and sensory stimulation disrupt the processes of the steady physiological state, homeostasis. Therefore, the first aim is to *supplement* the inadequate movement patterns of older people. Maslow calls this type of therapy *restoration therapy* (Maslow, 1962).

Many older people have developed the habit of inactivity. As a "habit is stronger than nature itself," it is usually difficult to overcome (James, 1962). But when the habit involved is that of inertia, it requires even greater force to reverse. Just knowing that some form of exercise is essential is not enough to change the habit. Therefore, the second principle is to *stimulate* older people to want to take this movement supplement. Here we become involved with the concept of motivation.

"Motivation is what impels us to certain things rather than others" (Bois, 1966). Enjoyment appears closely bound up with motivation. Sigmund Freud regards the "pleasure principle" as the decisive factor in behavior and the physiological psychologist James Olds has proved by laboratory tests on the hypothalamus

46

that we choose pleasure and avoid pain despite the strength of other motivations (Olds, 1971).

According to Abraham Maslow, motivation functions as a mechanism for fulfilling each of five basic needs. These are of varying intensities, depending on how fulfilled each need is at any given moment.These needs, in order of importance, are (Maslow, 1954):

physiological needs
security
belonging and love
recognition
self-development and congenial activity

The teacher or therapist who is aware of these needs stimulates the interest of the participants through the pleasure principle. As men and women begin to enjoy the satisfaction of participating in this new movement experience, they are further motivated to continue because many of their needs are met. The therapist fills these needs, in part, through the application of the "six s's." These principles shape the attitude and manner of the therapist or leader and establish the guidelines of the procedures in the following ways:

1. By fulfilling a *physiological need* through supplementary movement and sensory stimulation
2. By meeting the need for *security* through the physical safety of the movement in a chair and the psychological safety of the teaching methods
3. By building a supportive *feeling of belonging* through promoting a feeling of group identity
4. By *recognizing* each participant's unique achievements and accepting and accommodating their limitations
5. By relaxing the group. An activity with a group that

47

laughs easily at the same things is a *congenial activity*. As the participants develop and change their frame of reference from fatigue and depression to relaxation and exhilaration, their exercises become both significant and satisfying.

When any of the basic needs are poorly gratified, psychological aging is influenced adversely. Sensory deprivation resulting from impairment or loss of one or more senses causes much of the damage. The psychologist Donald Hebb is quoted as saying that there is a *psychological tonus* not much different from physiological tonus which is maintained by arousal stimuli. When these drop below a certain level of activity, all activities are affected (Kleemeier, 1964). It is essential then that therapeutic movement provide sensory stimulation to supplement the deficit.

Using these principles in our work with older people, we follow a structured yet expressive approach. The movement studies are composed within the structural limitations of the "six s's." This limits the form to seated exercises, but the possibilities for movement and sensory stimulation are endless. The participants experience these movements expressively, through their aroused kinesthetic sense, and react with pleasure and laughter and a feeling of power, sensitivity, and grace.

The therapeutic outcome of expressive movement has been widely known by primitive societies throughout history. In the 1930s, the biological mechanism for the prolonged and pervasive reaction to sensory stimulation in general was discoverd in the central nervous system. It is called the *ascending reticular arousal system* (ARAS) that "projects diffusely to thalamic, hypo-thalamic, and cortical regions" (Thompson, 1967). These are the regions in the brain where the awareness of pain and pleasure occur. The slow action of the ARAS gives delayed stimulation to these feelings and partly accounts for the prolonged periods of euphoria following movement sessions. Some comments from participating patients in a convalescent hospital may illustrate

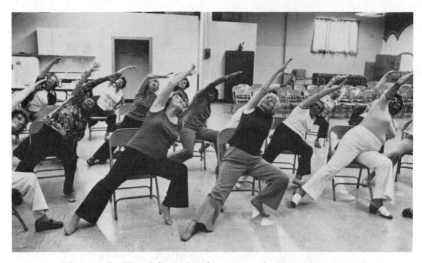

Figure 7. The kinesthetic sense: feeling the stretch

how the stimulated kinesthetic sense affects the patient's mood.

One man was heard to object loudly to being wheeled into the exercise room. After participating in a chain of hands that gently pulled him to and fro, he said, "I feel a surge of life!" Another tactile experience of receiving rhythmic pulsations through the hands elicited the comment, "It makes me feel secure." A stroke patient commented, after a slow, luxurious movement of the shoulders, "It makes me feel beautiful."

The sense of touch and the kinesthetic sense are most central to the psychological effect of the movement experience, but the senses of seeing and hearing also play a role. The participant sees the therapist demonstrate all the sequences and hears the verbal accompaniment of instruction. This method bypasses failing memory. When necessary, it also bypasses a vision or hearing deficit, since either sense can get sufficient information without the other.

The verbal instructions are similar to the instructions from an air traffic controller in a watchtower who "talks" a pilot down to the field in safety in a dangerous situation. They give the

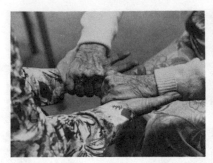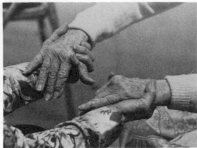

Figure 8a. A tactile experience of rhythmic pulsations: one person squeezes . . .

Figure 8b. The other person answers

participants the temporary use of an additional brain and of that brain's knowledge. Accordingly, the instructions form a constant stream of signals and cues. As gerontologist James Birren noted, "When appropriate cues are provided at the retrieval stage, difficulties of older people are reduced" (1972). In other words, the visual and oral cues supplement the information the participants retrieve from their own memory.

Movement Techniques

In accomplishing our goals, we use both relaxing and vitalizing techniques. Both methods are strengthened through a muscle awareness characteristic of the kinesthetic sense. The relaxing techniques are motor responses of giving in to gravity. The vitalizing techniques are achieved mostly through rhythmic movements opposing gravity (Humphrey, 1959). A few exceptions are the extremely mild and limited use of *isometric* contractions (Wells, 1966).

Both the vitalizing and the relaxing movements in relation to gravity, as developed in Doris Humphrey's theory of fall and recovery, have enriched the vocabulary of dance with terms and concepts well suited to the therapeutic movement for the elderly. *Fall, rebound, swing,* and *suspension* are movement responses to gravity. They are the most effortless ways of moving. Another

50

term, *succession*, is a pattern of coordinated movements that progress along adjacent muscles and joints. The moving parts must first be controlled individually before they can be moved sequentially. Such a maneuver requires considerable conscious involvement. A simple facial exercise can illustrate this experience: lift and then depress one eyebrow and then lift and depress the other eyebrow. Continue to alternate these movements rhythmically and smoothly.

Energetic bending and stretching exercises give variety to the movements. One way we achieve the feeling of energy is by *co-contraction* (Wells, 1966) which, like isometric contraction, involves the principle of resistance. However, in co-contraction the effort results in a powerful movement as opposed to a held position. Martha Graham's dance vocabulary identifies these co-contraction movements as *contraction,* while flexing, and *release*, while extending. John Martin, former dance critic of the New York Times, describes Graham's movements as seeking ". . . to center the body and integrate the movement . . . to evoke a heightened awareness" (Martin, 1946).

Relaxation through movement occurs in three ways:

(1) A true swing is relaxing. It is a sequence of fall, swing, and suspension. The fall is effortless and starts a momentum that can continue to swing up in the opposite direction, where the movement is held effortlessly for a split second in suspension before changing direction, and the fall starts again. Some falls involve rebounds that give additional energy to the upswing.

(2) Another way of releasing tension is through stretching. Stretching or elongating a muscle is a part of every natural movement. The muscles work somewhat like draw draperies. One cord always lengthens while the other shortens to open or close the draperies. This is similar to the principle of body mechanics called synergistic action, and accounts for the release of tension during the rhythmic movement of exercise.

(3) Relaxation can also result from a variety of breathing

51

techniques. These vary with the kind of concentration that is suggested. Emphasis may be placed on sensory awareness or the use of imagery; or attention may be focused on different methods of breathing or even different rhythms of breathing.

But there is a chronic condition of tension that cannot be therapeutically relieved by any of these methods. Edmond Jacobson, who pioneered experimental research on tension and relaxation, was the first to realize that even at apparent complete rest, muscles could still retain *residual tension*. He developed a technique for relieving chronic tension which he called *progressive relaxation* (Jacobson, 1929).

Progressive relaxation starts with the person lying comfortably on the back. Following a systematic sequence of all the voluntary muscle groups of the body from head to toe, the person tenses one muscle group and lets it go limp, and continues with the next until all the muscles have been relaxed in this way. As students experience the difference between a relaxed and a tense muscle, they can learn to recognize and relax unproductive tension. Moving with this kind of efficiency is called *differential relaxation* (Jacobson, 1929) and results in a greater capacity for activity without fatigue.

The above techniques are modified to the extent of effort or concentration that the participants can tolerate comfortably. They must be able to perform and experience all activities without pain or strain. The concept of *tolerance* (Logan and Wallace, 1964) which is modified to fit the capacities of the older person determines the duration, tempo, and intensity of the exercise sequences.

Energy

We must be careful of the kind of effort the older person is called upon to make. It appears that there are two kinds of human energy: the physical energy measurable and replenished by calories; and the mental energy of problem-solving that is not.

The first kind is expended in simple physical activity such as bending and stretching. The second kind is expended in psychological adjustments to new situations.

Hans Selye calls the latter *adaptive energy* and suggests the theory that we are born with a genetically determined amount of adaptive energy which can be used up in an exciting life or prolonged in a dull one. "Only when all our adaptability is used up will...death follow" (Selye, 1956). This sheds light on the reluctance of older people to enter into new experiences. It appears to be self-protective and due to a dwindling amount of adaptive energy.

Therapists must hold to a minimum the expenditure of adaptive energy required by participants to adjust to a class. Let us remember: physical energy must be spent; adaptive energy must be saved.

How much physical energy and strength can be realistically expected of older people? We can begin with the simple idea that "one must exert energy to move...(and that)...the range, intensity, duration, and speed of every movement are dependent on the output of the energy and force exerted" (Hawkins, 1965). If we choose, as an example, a sedentary person who sits all day, even the rhythmic turning of the head or elevation and depression of the shoulders eight times might represent a 400- to 800-percent increase of directed energy.

But the geriatric population includes the golfer and dancer as well as the wheelchair patient, and with people of different degrees of physical capacity between these two poles. We must take the cue from the *entering behavior* of the participants (De Cecco, 1968). The rhythm is taken from their walking tempo as they enter the room. The size and effort of these movements are gauged by their other normal gestures. This ensures, at the start, that the exercises will be within the tolerance of the participants.

Bear in mind that the stress of gravity on the participant is limited at the very outset, since all the exercises are done in a straight-backed chair. From this point on, all the movement is kept within the physical tolerance of the individual because:

1. The movement combinations and the sequence are arranged within the constraint of tolerance.
2. Most participants feel their own limitations and do not go beyond them.
3. The therapist learns to pick up subtle cues of fatigue, stress, impatience, disinterest, difficulty, and pain—or evidence of interest, pleasure, or interaction—and responds to the individual or group as a whole. With their physical and psychological safety protected, the participants can enjoy the dynamic group experience of the class without anxiety.
4. Where a participant approaches his or her own limits of exertion, the leader requests "resting this one out." This means the participant relaxes for the duration of the exercise.
5. Biofeedback experiences are introduced in community-based classes and classes that meet in retirement homes. The participants take their own pulse rate (Morehouse, 1975). Learning to find and count one's pulse on cue becomes an interesting activity as well as a safety check. Using Dr. Morehouse's method, the "average resting pulse" is taken before exercise and then compared with the "average action pulse" which is taken after the exercise. Comparison of the two pulse rates gives the students biological information about the efficiency of their own hearts in rest and activity.

As this is a group procedure, the therapist (or teacher or leader) gets the information as well, and acts accordingly. Most of the students become tired by the time their action pulse rates reach about 110. This is an increase of 30 to 40 pulse beats a minute for most of them. For reasons of safety, we avoid movement that pushes the pulse rate any higher.

Sociological Considerations

The psychological and physical constraints of GBD may differ from movement therapy of other age groups mainly in degree, but one constraint is uniquely important to the aging population: the therapist must be especially sensitive to the *semantic states* (Bois, 1966) of the participants. The current generations of older people have grown up in Victorian early twentieth century or pre-World War I times. Many still hold a restrictive attitude which affects their responses in body movement classes. It inhibits their ability to work with body image and parts of the body. For instance, early in the century modesty was a highly respected trait in women. Mention of any body part between the waist and the feet was considered unseemly, especially in mixed company. Legs were called "limbs." Knees were tightly pulled together in a seated position for fear of appearing suggestive.

To overcome this influence, the therapist employs two psychological techniques: motivation and semantics. Semantically, the metaphor that the body is a machine significantly changes students' attitudes toward their bodies; it instills a respect for the maintainance of their biological machines; and it depersonalizes their feeling about their bodies to the extent that they can begin to move inhibited areas with equanimity. (This approach is elaborated in Chapter 10.)

This respect for technology is further reinforced by an equal respect for medical authority.

Within a short period of a month or two, most women shed the taboos during the class and begin to experience appropriate responses to their movements. Then movement sensation and expression begin to work their magic.

Comparisons and Contrasts

The somato-psychic approach of GBD is midway between dance therapy and physical education. It shares similarities with dance therapy in its psychological emphasis on feelings. And it shares similarities with physical education in its somatic emphasis on body mechanics.

GBD aims to maintain or restore older people to health through vitalized movement and ventilated emotions. Like dance it is an expressive technique that yokes action and reaction of a movement into one total experience. But unlike many dance therapists who start with feelings, GBD instructors achieve this experience through the more objective approach of motion preceding emotion, i.e., you stretch—and you feel good (or bad as the case may be); you push—and you feel strong; you swing—and you feel free.

These movement sensations also kindle emotions by linkage to past events. They set off "reverberating circuits of association" (Hebb, 1966). A swinging movement hooks into youthful experiences that reinforce carefree happy feelings. Smooth movements reawaken gentle feelings. Percussive movements connect with feelings of assertion. Rhythmic movements revive buoyant whimsical feelings, and coordinated movements reawaken a feeling of grace.

These intuitive movements are a language of self-expression. Even though the participants are limited to the seated position, with this vocabulary they are able to ventilate feelings of anger, power, sympathy, fun, and friendship; emotions which are curbed or dormant in the authoritarian atmosphere of most long-term facilities.

If we compare GBD with adapted physical education, we see that both are concerned with the improvement or restoration of physical mobility. And both invest the mind in the body to coordinate its many parts. But GBD emphasizes the benefit of the sensation of the movement equally with the movement per-

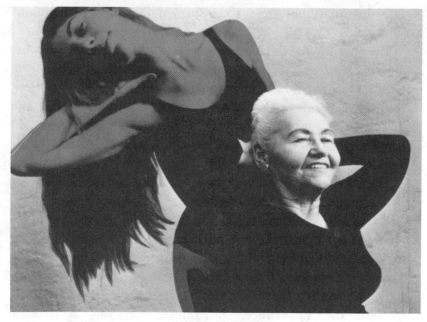

**Figure 9. Polly and Berdie: movement restores feelings of
our youth**

formance. This develops kinesthetic awareness. Physiological
aspects of this awareness gives us the body-sense that puts us in
touch with the "wisdom of the body." We learn to "read" the
body's messages which are coded in the muscles as degrees of
tension and relaxation. Reading movement has the same purpose
as reading a book; i.e., for information.

One of the insights gained is the relationship between muscular
tension and pain, e.g., "tension headache" (Brown, 1974);
another is between emotional tension and breathing. "Emotional
states and breathing patterns are very much interrelated ...
respiration patterns become irregular with anger, slow and
deepen with relaxation, and quicken in fear and stress" (Pelletier,
1977). "The relation between depressed mood and depressed
breathing is so direct and immediate that any technique which

activates breathing loosens the grip of the depressive mood" (Lowen, 1974).

The physiologist Edmond Jacobson was "convinced that many illnesses were social diseases of tension and that release from muscle tension could be therapeutic." He detected the "relationship between mind and muscles . . . emotion and muscles . . . and muscles and muscles" (Brown, 1974). He demonstrated that psychological or emotional stress is reflected in tension by the muscles.

These insights give us the physiological basis for the therapeutic changes that body-awareness and activity can effect. Body messages of tension, which in biofeedback laboratories are recorded in electromyograms, can also be decoded by the nervous system through the *sensori-motor circuit* (Brown, 1974). Tension messages of distress can be alleviated by relaxing, moving, and/or breathing techniques. Messages of painful stiffness can be reduced by gentle stretching and touch techniques.

Anxiety and depression can be alleviated by a variety of conscious breathing techniques. The group experience as a whole can promote therapeutic change for participants suffering from loneliness and boredom. Selye says "deviation is particularly important in combatting purely mental stress . . . you must find something to put in the place of worrying thoughts to chase them away." He defines deviation as "turning something aside from its course" and compares deviation to sublimation, a psychoanalytic term, which he defines as "the act of directing the energy of an impulse from its primitive aim to one that is culturally or ethically higher" (Selye, 1956).

Using Selye's principle of deviation, the original preoccupation with worry is diverted to the more pleasurable group exercise. At this point the pleasure principle operates as "nothing erases unpleasant thoughts more effectively than concentration on pleasant ones" (Selye, 1956).

In GBD all these ideas, methods, and results coalesce into benefits for the senescent student even during the simplest movements.

9

Teaching the Senescent Student

UNFORTUNATELY many people approach the role of student with misgivings and conflicts. Their divided feelings grow out of the antagonism between their attitudes and needs. They need to learn how to adjust to the changes of retirement and the aging process. Education can teach them new ways of coping with their waning capacities, but they may consider it a threat to their self-respect. Many aging people resent any situation that suggests they are inadequate or weaker than they once were.

The image of most older people in the United States is constantly attacked. Their personal influence is diminished by their separation from the mainstream of productive life. This social decrease of power is often paralleled biologically by deterioration of health, mobility, and appearance. To counteract this double-barreled assault, they may pass through endless and exhausting self-justification.

Often change itself is considered the culprit. Change has hurt them, and they react by affirming the rightness and goodness of all traditional attitudes, even those which no longer work ("if it was good enough for my father . . ."). This attitude reinforces the double-bind of their need for and yet aversion to the new ideas transmitted through continuing education and therapy.

How can we, as educators, therapists, and recreators who are agents of change, serve within this situation? All of us are ready and able to help the elderly increase their factual information, help them function better, and increase their opportunities for participating in more desirable activities. We know that these changes do occur when older people invest their energies in our programs.

But for the older person, becoming a learner instead of a teacher is to lose self-esteem. The trade-off of pride in knowledge for humility in learning may seem too high a price. As adults and parents, older people have grown accustomed to giving directions, not to following them; ordering, not obeying. In short, they may easily see schooling as an occupation for children and resent the implication of their "second childhood." Memorizing is likely to be particularly irksome because they have long been aware of their failing memory and fear its exposure.

A brief look at the dynamics of learning may help us. Admittedly, learning occurs on two levels. Quantitatively, we acquire masses of information; qualitatively, we reach a new level of understanding, a new state of feeling. When the learning experience results in the immediate qualitative change of feeling better, geriatric students discover, to their surprise, that their objections dissolve. They become curious about the other benefits that are presented and grow interested in attaining them.

This is *learning readiness*. Suddenly the student is willing to try new things and begins to grow. What follows is a spiraling sequence of motivation: curiosity, interest, attention, focus, discovery, surprise, and exhilaration.

Thus, we see that the first principle of convincing an older person to become a student is to *achieve the immediate result of feeling better*. But an interesting thing happens as teachers and therapists seek this qualitative change in their students. We, as teachers, change. When we want them to feel better as students, we begin to care more for them as individuals. As a result of this change, the second principle achieves itself. This personal rapport promotes a caring relationship instead of the authoritarian one that threatened the student originally.

Simple, But Not Simplistic

Assuming that the teacher has been able to solve these initial problems in starting a class, he or she is then faced with another paradox of the aging personality: often as physical capability diminishes so does mental ability, but the feeling of sophistication does not. As the student's capacity lessens, instructions must be *simplified*. Yet the sophisticated student recognizes and resents a simplistic approach.

The following transcription of a taped interview with an activity director reveals the classic situation in a convalescent hospital:

> .... I've set up a program doing about a half-hour of different exercises. I intersperse it with games with mental stimulation. I slow it down, and before we know it, it's time for lunch.
>
> So—my classes have grown from eight people to fifty. I need more room, and I need different sessions now. It's great! The members may not know my name, but they wait for me every morning when I come in. It's great, but it drains you. It drains you! And the hardest thing I find is to constantly come up with new things to do!
>
> You know, you don't want to introduce too many—or too difficult—things, because they can't handle it. Yet you don't want to keep the same thing all the time, because they get bored.
>
> It can't be too intricate, and it can't be too simplistic, because they catch on right away. "That's kid stuff," they say. "That's for children."

The problem here lies in the difference between the two words, *simple* and *simplistic,* which are intertwined. Theoretically, *simple* and *simplistic* are opposites. Simplistic thinking is a mechanical acceptance of an idea or act. The act is generally easy to imitate and leaves the doer uninvolved. In a simplistic presentation, the teacher is also uninvolved. S/he does not wonder about it, digest it, or grasp it. Instead s/he picks it up, accepts it, and hands it to others without understanding its meaning and function.

The word *simple* involves a different process. It is the result of extracting meaning from ideas and skills. When the purpose or meaning of an idea is understood, it becomes simple. Meaning makes the difference!

There is nothing simplistic about body movement. But without understanding, a direction lacks meaning. It is demeaning. This is the insult of the simplistic approach.

Even such a simple movement as bending and extending the fingers becomes a significant experience when it is taught with a sense of meaning or purpose. The teacher who understands this can inspire the student with the knowledge of the benefits each exercise provides.

For instance, at the start of a finger exercise the teacher may emphasize the improvement in circulation. During the following week he or she may stress the importance of stretching as a deterrent to contracture. Still another way to enhance interest is to focus attention on the *synergistic* action of complementary muscles, pointing out that one set shortens in contraction, or tension, while the other lengthens, releasing its tension.

The Pleasure Principle

Just knowing what is good for us does not always ensure its being done. Overcoming inertia requires additional incentives such as curiosity and pleasure. Any undertaking started in curiosity will certainly be continued, if it proves to be pleasurable.

The very idea of exercising in chairs is likely to provoke curiosity. People will come to see a class, but will they stay to participate? Yes, if they find it enjoyable as well. How can

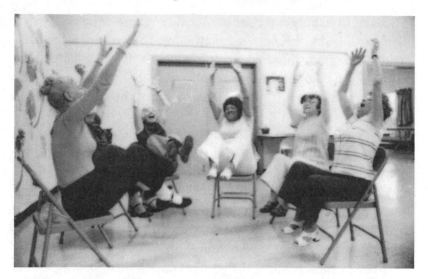

Figure 10. Instead of fatigue, there is exhilaration

physical exercise, normally considered uncomfortable and even painful, be undertaken happily?

Geriatric Body Dynamics is a unique program precisely because it eliminates the distressful aspects of exercise. Instead of tedium, there is discovery. Instead of pain, there is comfort. Instead of fatigue, there is exhilaration. Instead of threat, there is support. Instead of failure, there is success. Instead of atrophy, there is growth. Instead of awkwardness, there is grace. The students anticipate the class as a well-planned event that brightens the day's schedule. In intermediate and total care facilities, participation becomes a status symbol of self-dependence, while for healthier people it may be a transition to greater independence and activity.

One of the ways this program reduces the resistance to exercise is through the pleasure principle of aesthetics. Beauty is consciously employed as a catalyst to stimulate the older person to participate.

In fact, the whole exercise class is choreographically conceived. The participants become a functioning part of an artistically created ceremony that one might imaginatively call a "Ritual for Life." Even though the students may be unaware of the choreography, they fully enjoy the power of the whole aesthetic ritual.

Let us consider the "spectacle" of the class—the attractively attired students seated in a gentle curve of rows of chairs, the inspiring teacher image, the kinesthetic satisfaction of the exercises themselves, done in unison in the varying rhythms and qualities inherent in human movement. The entire lesson is governed by the aesthetic principles of form, unity, harmony, rhythm, variety, color, and content.

Through these means, the student experiences beauty and is part of the beauty. He or she becomes invested with a growing feeling of pride and conscious pleasure. The pleasure principle thus becomes a powerful lever for moving aging persons, contrary to their inclination, toward the vital physical activity of the exercise ceremony.

Visitors

Anyone who wishes to participate is always welcomed in the class. The only admission fee is participation. After all, visitors are potential students who are likely to be more skeptical than the rest of the class. They generally know they should participate, but are not sure that they can or want to. Shyness, lack of confidence, or reticence to participate in a new experience may hold them back. They may be lazy, depressed, or even disengaged. Whatever the cause, they are not prepared to commit themselves to this activity.

Curiosity has brought them to visit the class. Somehow, they hope that the "spectacle" will help them make up their minds. But a skeptic cannot be convinced to join the class until he or she becomes involved with the process and results of the exercises.

That is why the instructor helps visitors make a vital decision by insisting on the rule that all visitors sit with the group and participate in the class when they wish.

There are other reasons for this rule as well. The visitor who is observing uninvolved becomes an audience, and an audience implies performers. Performers are trained to divide their concentration between their actions and their audience's reactions. But Geriatric Body Dynamics is not a spectacle by performers; it is a ritual done by participants. The student who is conspicuously observed by a visitor during the class may become self-conscious and less involved in the actual exercise. The teacher's concentration is also divided by awareness of the observer's reactions.

The nonparticipating visitor not only distracts the class but also shatters its singleness of purpose. The guest may react to the unusual procedures in many ways. The exercise movements may seem strange and appear comical. The beneficial effects will dissolve if the class feels they are being laughed at—either during or after the session. It is only through the guest's participation that the purpose of the movement becomes evident. The exercises do not seem strange, bizarre, useless, or child's play to the visitor who experiences their beneficial results as a participant in the group. No participation, no visitation!

Group Dynamics

Group dynamics is a social force that deals with the power of a group to influence the individual. It is the flow of energy generated in a group which can influence the reactions of an individual and even release the reserve power of that individual to move with greater energy within the group. But what is this reserve power and where does it come from?

We think of human energy as physical force expressed through strength and endurance. But there are additional sources of power. The psychological power of motivation which involves one's inclination and desire affects the hormonal system and can increase a person's energy tenfold. A group that affirms and rewards individual action strengthens the individual's power to act.

A person may become involved in a group that works either constructively or destructively. If the members focus on hate or vindictiveness, we see the use of this power in a threatening way, as with mob violence. When the emotions of empathy and appreciation are in focus, these harmonious feelings inspire a release of individual power for self- and group-improvement and mutual enjoyment.

Human beings need group identification. Each person has a need to express herself or himself as a member of the group. But the difficulty lies in finding the right group and having the ability to express oneself in it. Efforts made at organizing group activities are only successful to the degree that this expression evolves; then group dynamics are set into motion. A collection of fifteen or twenty isolated people watching television in a recreation room still remains a collection of lonely individuals. But with a common activity in which they can express themselves through contact and interaction, that collection of people can quickly become a cohesive group.

Interaction with others for self-improvement becomes a constructive group activity. Movement is a very personal way of expressing oneself. Moving in rhythm with others gives one a sense of being part of a group. And moving in unison with others gives one a special sense of group identity. This "in group" feeling stimulates a sense of relationship and releases that kind of reserve strength that comes with being "in step." Energy increases with the confidence and conviction that one is doing the right thing.

A knowledgable leader who understands these dynamics can involve isolated individuals so that they function as a group. The teacher must first become aware of this process and then direct the group into a harmonious course. To be effective, the leader must create the conditions for *good humor of comradery, enthusiasm, exhilaration,* and *inspiration.*

Good Humor of Comradery

Because most people do not consciously express their feelings through movement, the opportunity to do so feels unusual. There are a lot of words for feeling unusual such as *strange, unexpected, zany,* or *funny.* When this emotion combines with a pleasant feeling, we begin to see the whimsical aspect of the situation. This puts us in a good humor; we become receptive; anything unusual becomes amusing. Laughter comes easily; and when laughter rises from mutual feelings in the group, it acts as a cohesive emotion that unifies a group. Laughter is a happy expression of the "in group" feeling that comes with group identity and comradery.

Enthusiasm

Emotions are infectious. The group is suggestible, and the strongest expression of an emotion affects the prevailing climate of the class. Will it be the skepticism of an aging adult or the enthusiasm of the teacher?

The instructor's enthusiasm is born of a conviction that: (1) the movement activity is an enjoyable experience; (2) the students can share the movement skills; (3) the students will benefit from the activity by experiencing a sense of well-being and by becoming more physically fit; and (4) physical fitness improves health and the ability to enjoy life as an alternative to an otherwise deteriorating existence.

Exhilaration

Rhythmic unison is the common denominator of the movement ritual. Contrary to the regimentation one usually associates with moving in unison, individual differences are accepted.

The teacher recognizes, and rewards with appreciation, the achievements made within the physical limitations of each student.

Rhythmic unison of the breath with the movements and/or sounds is the leavening influence of this exhilarating experience. Inhaling and exhaling more deeply with each movement improves the respiration. By getting more toxic air out of the body, more good air can come in; the feeling of heaviness dissipates and the aerated body feels lighter and freer and becomes more responsive.

Moving together, the whole class becomes one dynamic organism. Like one voice in a chorus, each participant enjoys the energy of the total group. Tapping this source of energy is exhilarating. This feeling continues to grow with the infectious freedom of carefree swinging movements and an increasing feeling of energy instead of fatigue.

Inspiration

A good teacher gives direction to this new feeling of animation and effectively guides the students toward greater physical improvement. But some teachers can influence their students' values by example, as well. They can stimulate a fuller appreciation of movement and they can function as a "role model."

The inspired student begins to see the teacher as a model which s/he wishes to emulate. This attitude works continually as a force for self-motivation. The new feeling is one of identification rather than competition. This step of identifying with the instructor helps students to bypass the pitfalls of embarrassment and awkwardness. Instead, they empathize with the skill and grace of the demonstrated movement and feel at ease with their own.

Finally, the emphasis on positive attitudes and the omission of negative ones provides the optimism in which the feelings of inspiration, enthusiasm, good humor, and exhilaration thrive.

The therapeutic value of optimism is very much a part of the holistic health movement and is being examined scientifically as a measurable characteristic.

In his book, *Optimism: The Biological Roots of Hope,* the anthropologist Lionel Tiger expresses the belief that the sense of a benign future acts as a survival mechanism, and reports that research in neurochemistry is currently involved with the possibility that there is a location in the brain for good feelings about the present and the future (Tiger, 1979).

People in the "helping professions" who consistently reinforce a climate of hope with their groups can confirm the improvement that occurs in the moods and behavior of their students/clients/patients. Not the least important effect of this group process is the group identification that serves to prevent or counteract "the isolation which later maturity creates day by day in ever increasing degree." Dr. George Lawton calls this form of therapy "maturity rehabilitation" (Lawton, 1956).

All the above motivational techniques have one aim: to entice the older person out of a cocoon of inertia and loneliness and into a pursuit of the physical, mental, and emotional stimulation essential to a sense of well-being.

The Role of Ritual

A *ritual* is a celebration of respect for life and the sources of life. It is established by consensus of the group and is performed in a predictable ceremony. The participants must believe in its importance. Every aspect of the ritual has meaning and purpose. The time, place, arrangements, equipment, attire, mood, purpose, and activity are established and repeated in the faith that, as every aspect of it becomes predictable, the desired outcome will also be predictable and inevitable.

It is in this sense that the movement sessions are a ritual—not to be confused with routine. Routine can become boring; ritual is inspiring. The purpose of a routine is to develop a habit through practice, so that the activity can be repeated accurately without thought. It frees the mind for something more important. Ritual celebrates the very importance of the practice by ceremoniously attending to every aspect of it.

The first class, and every other one to follow, is conceived as a ritual by the teacher and experienced as a ritual-for-health by the members of the class.

The First Class

The ritual starts with the scheduled *time* and *place*. The *equipment* is set up according to the floor plan. The teacher's image is established by his or her *attire*. The importance of the occasion is emphasized by the careful attention given to all the *arrangements.*

All these formal aspects of the ritual are repeated at every session. The day, time, and place are the same. The pattern of the chairs is the same. The students sit in the same places. The teacher's appearance is basically the same. The size of the group is generally the same. And the expectation of the reward of the ritual is the same. This anticipation of a therapeutic outcome, called the *placebo effect,* is part of the dynamics of the ritual. It makes each member of the group particularly receptive to the ritualized instruction.

The purpose of the ritual, of course, is always the same. It is a therapeutic group experience which promotes a beneficial change in the physical/mental being of each participant. The method is the same. It provides psychomotor and psychological stimulation through a series of familiar movement studies performed in a chair. It is followed by a guided discussion of the health-producing effects of one or more of the movement experiences. Together, the activity and discussion reinforce the expectation and the results.

The movement ritual begins with a statement, "Now that we are all comfortably seated, let's start our class with a wake-up and warm-up exercise." (Some teachers may prefer a different opening statement.) What follows is a *ritualized approach* to the movements. The movements are *choreographed* into *studies*. The *sequences* are fairly predictable. Deviations in the form of simplifications or variations are made developmentally. As the situation changes with progress, the teacher introduces variations in tempo, rhythm, and coordination.

The sense of ritual is maintained despite this kind of flexibility which is essential in a person-oriented framework. It allows for accommodation and growth while it maintains the predictable procedure.

Several principles guide the order of the studies. Physical effort versus physical tolerance determines the order and duration of the active and passive studies. Sensory awareness invests the passive studies with active interest. Emotional involvement adds energy to the active sequences.

After the warm-up and Basic Position, the ritual continues with a core group of movement studies that release the emotion-stored centers of tension in the neck and torso which inhibit movement. The pattern of the ritual which is established in the teaching tape, *Invitation to Exercise,* is practiced in every session of the first unit of study. The text of the tape is in the *Exercise Manual* along with other teaching tapes for more advanced work to match group readiness and teachers' preferences.

The ritualized group experience progresses through action and interaction to initiate the therapeutic process. As the students feel better, their attitudes become more trusting and confident. They permit themselves the time and concentration essential to the creative process of restoration.

10
The Body
as an Instrument

The human machine has the advantage over the
manufactured machine; whereas the latter wears
out with use, the former improves, provided it is
used within the principles of efficient human
motion.
— DR. WILLIAM SKARSTROM

ONE OF OUR goals is to motivate the aging person to "move within
the principles of efficient human motion." Toward this end,
students must be helped to view their own bodies objectively.

In the beginning, the instructor directs the student's attention
to the body as an instrument, an instrument for living, for
pleasure, and for work. This instrument, then, is equated with
other machines such as automobiles, washing machines, and
television sets. Having owned at least one of these, most students
are familiar with the importance of maintenance and repair and
know that prompt and regular care of even the smallest part of an
appliance is essential for its continuing efficient service.

Through this analogy, students begin to accept supplementary
exercise as significant in the upkeep and repair of their own
bodies. They then begin to understand that such attention to their
own needs is not selfish, but prudent; that the time and effort
spent in exercise improves the body's functioning immediately;
that *the body improves with use.* The psychological improvement
that follows results from a series of chain reactions.

Focus on the parts of the body where the movement occurs
intensifies the inner sensations of the movement. This is a skill
called *muscular innervation* and is the prerequisite of body-
awareness. Stimulation of the skin by touch augments this skill.

Together they develop body-awareness, the sensation of one's self. Self-awareness is the opposite of self-consciousness, for it leads to an improved self-image by concentrating on ability rather than inadequacy.

As men and women are freed from their self-consciousness and can focus on any part of the body without embarrassment, the instructor can move away from the mechanical image of the body as a machine or instrument and begin to view the body psychodynamically. Now the students can concentrate on the sensory and emotional feelings of the movement and put their muscular awareness to work.

Constructive Muscular Awareness

There are many kinds of muscular awareness. When we say our back feels tired, we are indicating an awareness of fatigued muscles in the back. When we feel a blow on the arm, the pain focuses attention on the hurt area. When we have gentle kneading sensations, as in massaging, we react with pleasurable muscular awareness. When we suffer from the intense and prolonged contraction of a quadriceps muscle, the cramp focuses our attention on the thigh area, and we try to get rid of the pain.

Unexpected awareness in the muscles has occurred to almost everyone who has prepared to lift a heavy weight and has almost fallen backward when the object proved to be only a fraction of the weight anticipated. This surprise presupposes a muscle preparation of which we are not even conscious and dramatizes the reality of independent muscle awareness.

These examples of muscular awareness demonstrate our ability to be conscious of surface stimulation as well as of internal muscle action. This is passive awareness. Something is happening to the muscles of which the individual is pleasantly or painfully aware. But this kind of muscle awareness, arising from our sensory nerves, is also essential to constructive muscular awareness, which is active. With constructive awareness, not only can one be aware of something happening to one's muscles through the sensory nerves, but the individual can also initiate the activity through the motor nerves which send information from the brain to the muscles.

All our muscles are "wired" for messages—*motor messages* sent from the brain into the muscles, telling them what to do, and *sensory messages* returning to the brain from these muscles, communicating how the muscles feel. This loop, the sensori-motor circuit, makes muscular innervation possible to all human beings whose nervous systems are intact. When applied consciously it becomes a skill that can tell any voluntary muscle to work or to relax. Some muscles are working when they should be relaxing, as in residual tension; and some relax when they should work, as in poor posture. Both these conditions can be present in different muscles at the same time. With skill, a person can feel that his or her muscles are misbehaving and correct the condition by using more efficient motion.

This ability is especially critical for older persons. By using more efficient movement they can increase their comfort and decrease their distress at the same time.

11

Communicating with Students

THE INSTRUCTOR works on two levels of communication—verbal and nonverbal. *Verbal communication* involves all oral instruction and includes rhythmic verbalization, the "say it" technique, semantic discrimination, and discussion. Nonverbal communication includes movement, the "mirror me" and "show me" techniques, contact, manual instruction, intonation, music, facial and body expression, imagination painting, sensory awareness, touch, pairing, laughter, kinesthetic awareness, empathy, and group dynamics. We shall discuss each of these techniques in turn.

Verbal communication combines language and nonlanguage elements. Language elements include the words, symbols, and structure of the language. Their effectiveness is best demonstrated by books, periodicals, and correspondence, where the words unmistakably deliver the entire message. Oral communication, on the other hand, delivers the message not only through words but also through the speaker's voice, expressions, and movements—the nonlanguage elements. Through the flexibility of the voice, the speaker unconsciously expresses both feelings and ideas.

For example, have you ever gleaned two messages from one communication? If they disagree, the intonation of their voices may suggest a different meaning from what the words indicate. We recognize these differences in flattery and sarcasm.

Intonation is the melody that expresses the underlying feeling of the speaker. A student reacts more to the melody of a message than to the words. Respect for the student will color the voice of every teacher who sincerely believes that the normally aging older person is an intelligent, important adult, capable of responding to instruction adequately. With this underlying conviction, the tone of voice of the instructor will be consistent with the verbal message of instruction and will never imply that the student is wrong, inept, or stupid.

When a student does not respond as expected to an instruction, the teacher's task is to express the instruction in another way. Let us look at the many options.

Verbal Communication
Rhythmic Verbalization

Rhythmic verbalization is the audio part of the audiovisual demonstration method, in which the student hears as well as sees the instruction. The words provide meaning, and the voice of the instructor adds a pleasant percussive accompaniment which rhythmically beats out the movement and breathing directions. This technique is employed on all the *Movement is Life* tape cassettes.

By combining the demonstration of the movements and rhythmic verbalization, the teacher relieves the student from remembering directions, movement, sequences, and coordinations. This full presentation frees the student to concentrate on innervation during the movement and to enjoy the sensations of muscular vitality.

True muscular awareness is generally found in advanced or professional dancers or athletes. It takes a high degree of coordination and concentration to be able to coordinate, remember, and feel movement all at the same time. Rhythmic verbalization (along with the "mirror" and "show me" techniques discussed below) makes this quick leap into advanced muscular awareness possible.

"Say It"—Student Verbalization

"Say it" is an instruction to the students to repeat the specific words of instruction as they move. This technique is often used

during a more complex coordination. It is based on the axiom that there can be only one thought in the brain at one time. By speaking the very words of instruction, the student is forced to concentrate more fully on the mental part of the action. The mental part which directs the speaking organizes the action as well. It then becomes easier to coordinate the rest of the bodily action with the more easily-mastered speech. At first only the braver ones "say it," and as a chant develops, the rest join in. The students make the correct movement because it is *thought* correctly and it is *said* correctly. Consequently, it is also *done* correctly.

To use this technique effectively, the instructor must eliminate all nonaction words and all action words must be understood. When the students "say it," they do it; and it becomes almost impossible to move differently from what the instructions say. When they say "Arm, let go," or "Tighten buttocks," they concentrate on the part that moves and focus on the way it moves. This results in a well-innervated movement.

Semantic Discrimination

Some words—like *sunshine, luxury, love,* and *laughter*—make us feel good. Their opposites—*darkness, poverty, hate,* and *anger*—make us feel bad. But what about the word *senescence?* Instead of seeing it as a crowning reward of an additional 25 years of life and freedom, many people fear aging as a period of senility. Fortunately, attitudes can and do change. When we can restore the meaning and feeling of a satisfying life to the word *senescence,* we may be able to reduce some of the anxiety that is so injurious to older people.

Semantics is the study that deals with the meanings of words and changes in their meanings with usage. Our concern here is not so much with the actual meanings of the words as with our students' reactions to them. Therefore, we carefully select those words that will have the most therapeutic effect.

77

The instructor exercises semantic discrimination in the words used to project an idea, specifically avoiding commands and other words ordinarily used in a regular calisthenics class (including "counting to keep the rhythm") and ideas that tend to confuse or distract students. For instance, the instructor *avoids* directions on how *not* to do a movement.

Semantic discrimination discourages talking that is unrelated to the movement experience. It cuts away negative thoughts. Only the positive and constructive are emphasized in verbal instruction. The instructor uses words, phrases, and ideas that have either pleasant associations or no previous association.

Classes should avoid such words as *don't, wrong, right* and *left, bad, sick, tired,* and so on. Instructors must always avoid censure of any kind (even in intonation) as well as comparisons that imply censure, or public personal correction. They will be careful to mention the student's name only when approval and recognition are indicated.

Names are important! Learning the names of the students is one of the teacher's first duties. In therapeutic movement classes our interest in the names of our participants goes beyond the practical use of names as labels, because the names distinguish each personality. We are interested in the *feelings* aroused by the names. To each person the most evocative word in the whole language is his or her own name. The exchange of names by individuals signals the beginning of a relationship.

Let us start with the participant's surname, the official name, the name that commands respect. This is the family name, the name of the citizen—the name that carries the responsibility, credit, reputation, and material wealth. It is the name invested with dignity, the public name. Everyone has the right to address adults by their surnames. When we want to emphasize these more formal aspects of the personality, we address people by their surnames.

The given, or "first," name, by contrast, is private, personal, and special. It is full of emotional power. The memories of infancy and childhood permeate the given name. Voices have impregnated that name with their love and anger, threats and promises. The use of the given name is a privilege that must be earned.

In relating to the people of our groups, the sensitive use of both names has therapeutic possibilities. Initially, respect is expressed by learning and using the surname. As the leader demonstrates a genuine interest in the individuals of the group by word and deed, the occasional use of the first name stimulates alertness and warmth.

Men and women of a group feel confidence in their teacher in direct proportion to the immediate feeling of improvement that results from the class. By recognizing and applauding each participant's improvement, the teacher creates a channel of rapport. Once this channel is established, the first name becomes a tool which helps to build confidence, relaxation, good humor, easy laughter, and the desire to please.

When these feelings are stimulated authentically they promote therapeutic improvement. Good humor cancels resentment. Confidence cancels skepticism. Relaxation cancels tension. Laughter cancels anxiety. And all these cancellations of negative emotions are necessary to permit the healing processes essential to restoration or maintenance of health.

When a teacher's interest in his or her students is not genuine, the voice lacks conviction. At such times, the familiarity of first names is resented and becomes counterproductive. But the appropriate use of first names is like a secure embrace. It implies protection from censure or harm. It releases youthful feelings of pleasure and energy in response to the experience at hand.

Discussion

The last 15 minutes of the class may be devoted to information on class procedures, general questions, and private personal corrections. The more formal guided discussion period is introduced after the individuals have begun to relate to each other as a group. Chapter 13 treats the discussion period in depth.

Nonverbal Communication

Mastering the verbal skills—written and oral—is considered critical in our educational system. Although we absorb much of our information from nonverbal behavior, educators tend to overlook nonverbal cues as a form of communication. In our teaching practice we emphasize the power of nonverbal messages particularly through eye contact and touch. We have seen the vitalizing effects of the touching of hands, the meeting of eyes, and the meaningful gesture. Accordingly we employ several nonverbal techniques.

Movement

The *movement,* as demonstrated by the teacher, is the most important nonverbal form of instruction. The teacher demonstrates the exercise continuously and is a constant example of what to do. The movement experienced by the student is the basis for physical and mental awareness. "All sensation, all perception is dependent on movement" (Lowen, 1958).

"Mirror Me"

"Mirror me" is the instruction to the student to reflect the direction of the movement, as demonstrated by the instructor. The student reflects the direction of the demonstrated movement just as a mirror would. It also influences the student to use the demonstrated movement as a model.

By mirroring the teacher, the students are relieved of the responsibility of remembering what to do and in which direction to go. With this technique teachers can bypass confusing non-action words like right side and left side. It also avoids the monotonous effect of counting. This leaves the students free to concentrate on the sensational experience of the movement.

As we have seen, at first the students reflect the teacher's movement. Then the situation changes. As they become familiar with the exercises they begin to see the teacher's fluent movement as a reflection of their own feelings of strength and flexibility.

"Show Me"

"Show me" is the phrase that initiates a tactile response. In response to the request, "show me," the student indicates the location of the movement experience. They touch the area if it is small or firmly stroke the area to indicate a larger one. This touch and pressure on the external area intensifies the student's feeling of the internal muscular activity.

This awareness is the mental investment that makes the movement personally significant. It is an especially valuable device to use when students' attention starts to wander.

How does the direction, "Show me," work? Suppose the

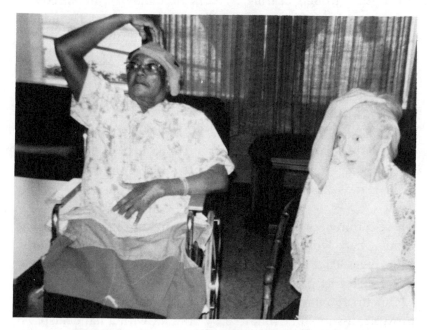

Figure 11. Exercise to achieve Basic Position

students have been asked to sit in Basic Position (see the *Exercise Manual,* Table I-A, Exercise 15). As their navels press against the spine, the students become aware of the whole abdominal wall. Upon request to "show me," they indicate the lower curve of the abdomen, with both hands touching the area of the abdominal wall. This focuses their attention on the relation between the movement and the location of the sensation. Actually touching the area with both hands intensifies the feeling by innervating the skin in the area as well. Achieving this feeling through touch bypasses much verbal explanation.

Contact

Contact is the most instant form of communication. Such meanings as *gentle, firm, encouragement, discouragement, punishment, support, like, dislike, good,* and *bad* are understood directly through bodily contact. The meanings do not have to be processed through hearing by ears that may be impaired, or interpreted by a mind that may be confused. Instead, students will feel what is directly perceived as pleasurable ("good") or painful ("bad").

Bodily contact is used in manual instruction. Of course, the teacher uses his or her hands sensitively. At least three degrees of pressure are employed:

1. Hands barely touching—sensitive hands.
2. Hands exerting the slightest pressure—comforting hands.
3. Hands clasped firmly together—capable hands.

These differences in pressure are developed in the instructional tape, *Once More-With Feeling* (see *Exercise Manual,* Table II-A, Figs. 30a & b). Both the instructor and the students develop this control as part of their action and interaction.

Our first contact with each person is with the eyes. Wherever possible, it should be followed by contact with a handclasp. As the class progresses, the teacher shifts eye contact from one

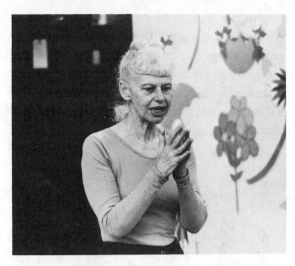

Figure 12. Hands barely touching

person to the other and varies observation of the facial expression with observation of the rest of the body movement. In this way, a teacher can scan the responses of each student. Some students require additional guidance through manual instruction.

Manual Instruction

Manual instruction requires individual attention. The teacher approaches a seated student. The student's awareness, initiated by self-touch in response to "show me," is further intensified during manual instruction, because another person's touch is more stimulating than one's own. Manual instruction is used sparingly, however, as the teacher can work with only one student at a time. Since the whole class must continue to exercise, it takes considerable skill for a teacher to motivate the rest of the class, while giving manual direction to one person. Many teachers use a tape to act as a surrogate teacher for the class while they concentrate on the individual instruction.

With experience, however, the teacher can approach one student while verbally continuing to instruct the whole class. He or she gently touches, taps, lifts, or presses the student in the area of the body involved in a specific exercise. The purpose of this manual direction may be to correct the movement unobtrusively or to emphasize for the individual the movement sensation to be felt in a particular area. Figure 13 illustrates the sensation of pushing against the teacher's hands to sense the action in the lower back.

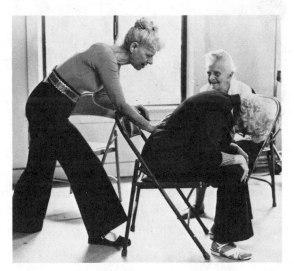

Figure 13. Stimulating body-awareness through touch and pressure — "Push my hands with your back "

In working with an unsighted or otherwise handicapped student, a teacher may ask the student to feel the teacher's movement, as in putting his or her hands on the teacher's shoulders to sense the extent of the shoulder's lifting. This caring instruction further enhances the students' experience by communicating a tender concern as expressed through gentle contact by the instructor. To be effective, manual direction must be carefully and appropriately used. This establishes the tone of the interpersonal relationships that are developed in the more advanced pairing exercises. If the exercise warrants it, the teacher may continue to move to other individual students until he or she has given half the class some manual instruction, and then promise to work with the other participants during the next session.

Intonation

In instruction, *intonation* continues where contact leaves off. The flexible use of the voice provides encouragement, warmth, and humor. It also carries special meanings. (Examples of voice color and flexibility are found throughout the instructional tapes.)

Through voice flexibility, the lower register is used for bearing down; the upper register, or rising intonation, signifies upward push or lift. Smooth and sharp accents dramatize movement. The *ssss* sound during exhalation emphasizes smooth continuous movement. The *huh,* or sharp exhalation, emphasizes percussive movement. Each teacher will develop his or her own special intonations to communicate with the class.

Whatever the specific style, voice flexibility ensures variety and avoids droning. It also reveals the quality of feeling that the teacher has for the individuals of the group.

Music

The sound and quality of *music* is tremendously effective in changing behavior by modifying the emotions. The art of music is not only humanizing, it is also healing.

One of the important uses of music is to establish a desired mood or to change from a negative one. Marches have energy and brighten the mood. Waltzes have a relaxing and quieting effect. These ideas are developed in the book *Marian Chace: Her Papers* (Chaiklin, 1975) and in a music therapy book, *Music and Your Mind* (Bonny, 1973).

In our work, music is used as one of many tools and always with a specific purpose:

1. Music may be used to create a specific mood before the

class starts or at the conclusion of the lesson.

2. Singing one tone after each inhalation is a pleasurable device to increase the exhalation time of breathing. Singing is enjoyed as self-accompaniment to a movement phrase and increases the expressive experience of the exercise.

3. Music is one of the methods we use to develop sense memory. The auditory sense is stimulated by recalling the melody of a familiar song. The melody is heard silently in the students' minds. For example, the instructor may write the title of a familiar song on the blackboard: "Wedding March: Here Comes the Bride." The members of the class are asked to close their eyes and hear the melody in their minds. Or they may use the silent melody as a point of departure for other sense memories. The instructor can exercise the visual memory ("What picture comes to mind as you hear the 'Wedding March'?") or the kinesthetic memory ("Try to feel as if you are actually moving in that scene").

   A good example of breathing, singing, and the sense memory is found in the recording, *Think With Your Body/Feel With Your Mind* (see the *Exercise Manual*, Table III-A Exercise 20).

4. Compositions may be used to evoke ethnic, sensuous, spiritual, or other specific associations.

5. Music is also employed to enhance the emotional quality of the movement. All the instructional recordings in this program use music in this way.

6. The use of different compositions for the same movement increases the opportunities for variety. Rocking to the music by Mahler in *Think With Your Body/Feel With Your Mind* is a different experience from rocking to harmonica music country style in *Chair Skwairs*.

7. Music to impart energy.

It is also important to realize that music can be counterproductive. For instance, people who have hearing aids cannot filter out unwanted sounds. They can hear a voice clearly. They can hear music. But when music and voice are combined, the sounds become confused. Consequently, when instruction is important, music must be eliminated.

Similarly, the skill of innervation requires single-minded concentration on a specific set of muscles. Music enhances the total emotional feeling of the movement but interferes with specific focus. As a result, music must be eliminated from exercises developing the skill of innervation.

Remember, too, the power of the rhythmic signature and tempo of music. Indeed, one of the purposes of using music accompaniment is to keep movement in time with it. But for this very reason it can be harmful. The dictatorial effect that recorded music has on the tempo or the phrasing may undermine the safety of the exercise. The teacher may relax his or her responsibility to monitor the stress of the movement and be carried away with the speed, swing, energy, and flow of the music.

One final potential danger exists for the instructor who may be an excellent therapist, activity director, or teacher, but has a poor sense of moving to the rhythm of the music. The annoyance such an unmusical experience can cause among many of the students can be just as harmful as the stress they came to class to alleviate.

In working with the musical accompaniment provided by the cassettes accompanying this program, remember that the recorded lessons present only the audio part of a normally audiovisual experience. The aesthetic quality of the demonstrated movements cannot be transferred to the tapes. Therefore, we must rely on the music to express the aesthetic quality of the movement that cannot be seen.

The use of music in the instructional recordings is a compromise. Teachers should feel free to interrupt sequences once they have learned them. In this way the teacher can adjust movements to a slower or faster tempo when needed and can pause to emphasize muscular innervation during the movements.

It is helpful to use a rhythmic instrument for variety. Castanets are a good solution. The sound is pleasant and the teacher is free to demonstrate the movement while playing the rhythm. Playing the castanets is a skill and playing them while teaching takes additional practice.

The teacher who is fortunate enough to have a pianist must choose a person who is experienced in accompanying movement. Such a musician has either memorized a large repertory of compositions based on dance rhythms or can improvise in appropriate rhythms, and can pay more attention to the tempo of the movement and the needs of the teacher than the written instructions of the composition and the technical skill on the keyboard.

Music, when used judiciously, is a powerful tool for motivation and inspiration.

Facial and Body Expression

The instructor who enjoys moving projects an animated facial expression and encourages students to enjoy the exercises. The teacher's quip that "your smile is the price of admission" usually gets results.

Teachers also realize the importance of observing the students' facial expressions. They interpret the flush, pallor, or undue change of facial expression as a signal and are alerted for the safety of the student. When there is reason for concern the teacher directs the student to sit quietly in the basic postural position.

But what about body expression? Movement that expresses feelings serves three purposes: it (1) fills the need for physical movement, (2) provides opportunity for emotional release, and (3) shows how the student feels about doing the movement.

Remember, however, that an activity that emphasizes self-expression must permit individual differences. Respect for differences in individual needs and abilities is essential to the development of self-awareness and freedom of self-expression. The teacher who is concerned with a right or wrong method destroys the climate of self-discovery.

Similes and metaphors stimulate the imagination and free the impulse to move. Instructors can ask their students to move "as if" they were the flower, velvet eagle, or butterfly of the metaphor:

slow as a flower turning toward the sun
smooth as velvet
fly like an eagle
touch as delicate as butterfly wings
strong as a giant
stretch as if every bit of space you reach will belong to you

A metaphor is a verbal picture that evokes feelings. It is a device to reach emotional expression. You can think up your own metaphors or use poetry, plays, songs, novels, or the Bible as a resource for images that can be expressed in movement. Here verbal communication stimulates a nonverbal response from the students.

Imagination Painting

Imagination painting is a creative use of visualization. A small percentage of students claim they lack the ability to visualize; but most men and women, responding to the barest verbal suggestion, can visualize a scene and enrich the picture with their own happy memories. As they create the scene, they relive and enjoy it.

Imagination painting starts in a seated position, eyes closed, arms lifted, hands clasped behind the head, with slow, rhythmic breathing. The breathing is relaxed, because the uplifted arms enlarge the chest cavity which makes breathing easier. The closed

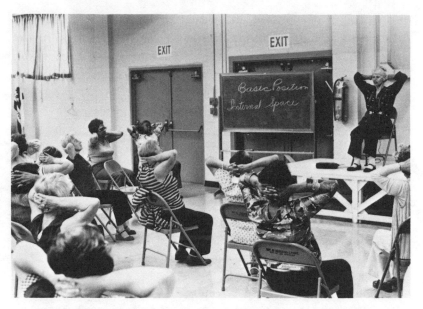

Figure 14. Imagination painting: hands clasped behind head

eyes cut out distractions and add to the feeling of relaxation and privacy.

A good example of this exercise may be found on the recording, *Invitation to Exercise* (see the *Exercise Manual,* Table I-B, Exercise 19). The suggestion is "blue sky, white clouds, shiny ocean, distant horizon." The image develops to the rhythm of the students' breathing and continues to grow as they are asked to paint anything else they wish into the picture. They may drop their arms any time during the exercise.

After about three to five minutes of visualizing, people are usually ready to open their eyes. Then comes the verbal part of the experience. At first, one or two of the most likely people are asked to share their images with the class. Sometimes the members are shy, at other times they are eager. The teacher encourages them all to express their feelings—but without pushing them to do it.

The sharing serves the purpose of self-expression. But the

teacher must constantly gauge the attention span of the rest of the class. S/he must balance the need for self-expression with the importance of maintaining class involvement.

The imagination painting interlude often follows a rather long or strenuous combination of movements. It serves as a restful activity between more strenuous exercises.

Sensory Awareness

Involvement in sensory stimulation by touch, balance, movement, visualization, and sense memory makes even the smallest movement significant. The simplest movements are appreciated when they are connected with mental stimulation. For example, consider the basic movement of rocking on the hips. As most of the exercise period is spent in a seated position, it is essential that the hips be relieved of the body weight repeatedly by this exercise, during every class.

Rocking can be repeated as often as needed, each time with a different emphasis. The teacher can emphasize circulation, changes in balance, holding, or whatever seems appropriate at the time. At first the students will be interested by the novelty of rocking. When the participants are ready for more input, teachers can begin to interlard the instruction with additional cues. They may ask, "Show me where you feel the movement. How does it feel?"

Another session may focus on changes in balance. "Lean to one hip. Where is the weight? Feel the air under the lifted hip. Show me, with your hands, where you feel the power holding you in this position." First you focus attention on the location of the holding, and then describe the feeling.

Verbal expression of the many different sensations wraps these discoveries into a neat, easily remembered package. Feelings which are put into words are more easily remembered. They provide the mind with a tangible framework for recapturing these feelings. This is part of the process of developing the kinesthetic sense.

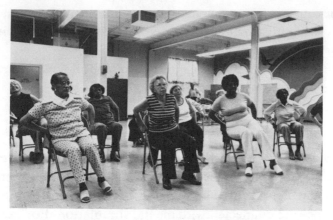

Figure 15. "Lean to one hip "

The instructor stimulates interest in simple movements such as rocking by introducing a variety of movement sensations:

1. *Rhythmic variety:* Changing the rhythm of the side-to-side rocking movement to three rocks and a hold. The hold arrests the movement and produces a strong kinesthetic contrast.

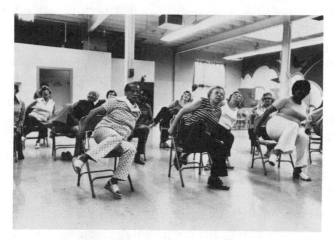

Figure 16. Rock with hold

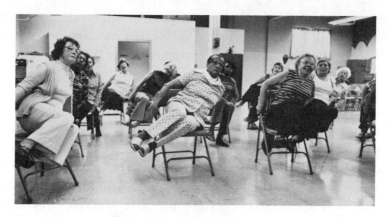

Figure 17. A feeling of fun

2. *Imagination:* Using an "as if" image. "Rock as if you are on a ride at Disneyland." This stimulates a feeling of fun.
3. *Pairing:* Having students hook elbows with the person next to them and then rock. This introduces the pooling of energies in the same rhythm for the same purpose.

Sensory variations such as these multiply the possibilities of enjoying the same fundamental movements with renewed interest. By combining sensation, movement, and understanding, the exercise, though simple, is not simplistic.

Touch

The simplest movement becomes fascinating when it is tied to the sense of touch. Let us repeat the exercise to develop sensitivity. Ask students to "Place both hands in front of you, palms facing. Gently and slowly move the palms toward each other. See how close you can get them without touching. What do you feel?" Repeat this maneuver a few times. Move them together and separate them. Finally, let them barely touch. "How does it feel now?"

We are performing on two levels of mental involvement—*action* and *reaction*. The act of moving the hands together and

93

apart is the result of psychomotor control. The reactions to the attraction of the hands toward each other—i.e., perceiving the warmth, the pull, and the vibrations—these are the result of sensory awareness.

The brain is bombarded by messages coming and going. The motor nerves are controlling the messages going to the hands. The sensory nerves carry the messages coming from the movement, warmth, vibration, and contact. The brain continues to be active with emotions such as pleasure at the gentle contact.

This elementary use of touch can be developed. Change the touch to slight pressure, strong pressure. Hold the hand of another person, alternating pressure and relaxation. Students can communicate through these pressures, so that one person pulses (squeezes lightly) and the other person answers:

"How does it feel?"
"It feels like I am not alone."

Each of these simple movements requires *attention, control,* and *awareness*—three mental processes. This kind of intellectual stimulation leads to self-awareness and awareness of others. This starts a friendly interaction among the students that is further developed in pairing.

Pairing

Pairing can be used in many exercises, and always involves two people relating to each other. This method of sensitive contact is generally employed to clarify or intensify a movement feeling. It is also used to reduce tension.

In classes where the people are ambulatory, both members of the pair may stand or one may stand and one sit. Many exercises are done with both members seated. Where there is a choice, men and women like to be paired together.

In the following studies, one of the partners, the *agent,* stands, while the other partner, the *subject,* sits. For clarity and

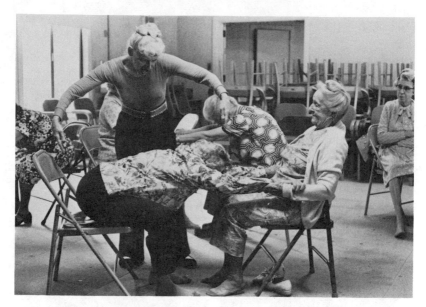

Figure 18. Intensify the feeling of stretch in the back

simplicity, we refer to the agent as "he" and the subject as "she," although, of course, the roles are reversed so that each person can benefit from the seated position.

The agent uses one of several possible motions: *touch, press, grip, stroke,* or *hold.* Following are some of the exercises and the purposes for which they are used.

Centering. The agent stands in front and a little to the side of the subject. The subject leans forward, in the Position of Relaxation (see Fig. 18). The agent makes contact with the subject's back by bending forward and lightly pressing his hands at the base of the spine near the coccyx. With both thumbs, he slowly draws two imaginary lines upward along both sides of the spine until the fingers stop at the base of the skull. The agent moves in a continuous motion to define the center of the subject's back. The subject senses this center line along the spine and is able to

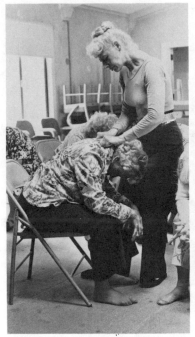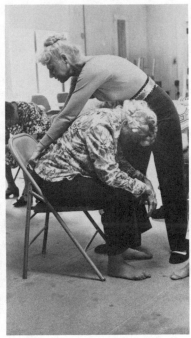

Figures 19a and 19b. Feeling of Center. The subject (seated) is experiencing a stimulating sensation along the spine by the gentle impression made by the (standing) agent's hands

identify the feeling every time the word *center* is used in relation to the spine. This feeling combined with Basic Position establishes the spine as the central core of the body.

The subject is also encouraged to relate subsequent movements to this feeling of *center*. The awareness of "the center" helps students follow an instruction of direction as well. For example, the instructor might say, "Gently draw your shoulder blades toward the center and let go."

Breathing. For this exercise, the agent, standing behind the subject, touches the area between her shoulder blades with both hands. This contact intensifies the subject's awareness of this area while breathing. The agent holds the position with slight pressure

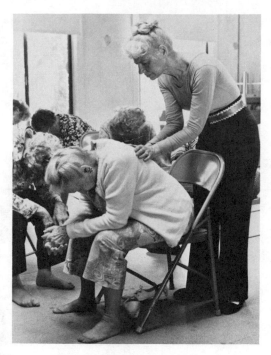

Figure 20. Breathe in. Send the air to your back between the shoulder blades

to intensify the subject's awareness of the expansion and relaxation of her back as she inhales and exhales. This technique helps develop costal breathing and is introduced in more advanced classes where the members have become accustomed to the sensitive use of touch and have interacted in other ways. (Costal breathing causes the rib cage to enlarge to allow more space for the lungs to inflate.)

Neck Pressure. A therapeutic technique, this exercise helps to alleviate the neck pain which can inhibit participants from the normal rotating or tilting action of their heads. The subject puts her hand on the side of the neck that feels tight or tense. The agent puts his hand on the same place, as the subject removes her hand.

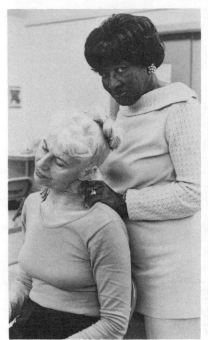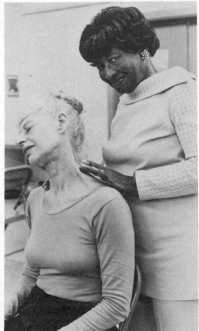

Figure 21. The agent grips the muscle as the subject tilts her neck

Figure 22. The agent grips the muscle as the subject rotates her neck

As the subject tilts her head to the side, the agent gently grips the contracted muscle (sternocleidomastoid muscle) of the flexed (short) side. The agent releases pressure as the subject rights her head back to center. If the subject's neck feels tight on both sides, then the pressure is alternated, first as the head tilts and bends to one side and then as it tilts to the other side.

After a few repetitions, the partners change positions. The sitters stand to become the agents, and the standers sit and become the subjects. In this relationship, the partners are interacting therapeutically. As the subject with the tight neck muscles feels the pressure of the other person's hands, her attention goes to the pressure instead of the pain caused by the tense muscle. The awareness of pressure reduces or cancels the awareness of pain, and the subject becomes willing to move the neck without fear. This maneuver may also be applied while the neck is rotating instead of tilting.

In any kind of movement the bending of a muscle, the *agonist*, involves the stretching of the muscle on the opposite side, the *antagonist*. This *synergistic action* which requires one muscle to stretch in order to allow the opposite muscle to contract is nature's way of keeping the muscles free of undesirable tension.

To see this action occur, just look in a mirror, tilt your head to the right, and watch the shape of the neck change. The neck seems shorter on the right side where the muscle contracts and longer on the left side where the muscle stretches.

When stiffness inhibits this natural movement, rhythmic exercise can generally regain the natural flexibility. But when pain inhibits this normal exercise then the therapeutic use of pressure is added. In this way the repeated stretching relieves the tension in the muscle while the improved circulation feeds the muscles in pain.

The therapeutic principle of combined movement and pressure can be explained to the students schematically, perhaps on a chalkboard. The schema for relieving a stiff neck is as follows:

The Situation: Tension + Pain + Inaction = Stiff Neck
The Therapy: Stretch + Pressure + Movement = Relief
The Method: Stretch cancels tension,
                pressure cancels pain,
                movement cancels inaction,
                relief cancels stiffness.

Neck Tension: Sometimes pain caused by muscular tension is experienced more on the stretch side of the neck. In this case, relief can be experienced by coordinating a light slow stroke along the path of the tense muscle on the stretch side. Start with two fingers behind the ear and continue to stroke the full length of the muscle to the tip of the shoulder joint. The slow, smooth, gentle stroke initiates a feeling of relaxation that is mimicked by the painful muscle. Whether students work alone or in pairs, the movement induces the muscle to "let go" and relax.

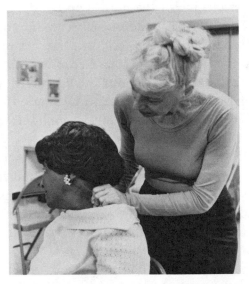

Figure 23. Stroking movement on stretch side

If we recognize pain as a physical signal for attention, then we can expect that getting that attention can be a psychological signal for relief. This describes, in part, the therapeutic result of the "placebo effect" of pairing. The other major aspect is touch, "tactual soothing which calms" (Montagu, 1972).

Kinesthetic Awareness

Movement experience and the memory (recognition and recall) of this experience are skills of kinesthetic awareness. We develop this skill in two ways: first, by becoming conscious of normal movements and circumstances, and then by changing inept movement responses and undesirable circumstances. To develop these skills participants learn to sense the following:

1. Voluntary tension (contraction) and release (stretch)
2. Voluntary relaxation
3. Non-voluntary residual tension
4. Weight distribution
5. Gravitational pull
6. Coordination
7. Body position

This process develops the sensation of the body-as-a-whole or body-awareness. Kinesthetic awareness is body-awareness in action. All the contact techniques, "show me," manual instruction, and pairing, are devices to excite this neuro-muscular awareness.

Many people think of the kinesthetic sense as the sixth sense, and like the other five senses, it is educable.

Empathy

Empathy is the internal sensation of an outside occurrence. Empathy enables us to identify with another person's expression of feelings as well. We feel like crying when we see someone cry; we feel like laughing when another person laughs. "It is this which provides the ultimate in psychological safety . . . if I see you and what you are feeling and doing . . . from your point of view and still accept you then this is safety indeed" (Rogers, 1961).

A personal interest has to be established between ourselves and others before there can be such a pathway of shared feelings. In class, after a mutual interest between students and teacher develops, such a relationship begins to grow. As the students empathize with the teacher, they can experience the movements of the teacher without awe or envy. They can identify with the teacher's energy and fluency as if it were their own.

Laughter

Laughter is communication, behavior, feeling, and therapy all in one. It feels good, is good, and does good at every level. Psychologically, laughter is the perception of humor or pleasure in a situation. Physically, it is achieved through the relaxation of the diaphragm, the throat, and other muscles of respiration. At the feeling level, laughter releases emotional tension by relaxing the very areas where tension builds up, in the chest and throat. Socially, laughter is a group mechanism for defusing a situation that could be tense.

Henri Bergson, French philosopher and psychologist, in his essay on *Laughter* maintains that tension and flexibility are two forces essential to the health of the body and mind. Inflexibility in either body or mind causes illness.

> Society . . . (is) suspicious of all inelasticity of character, mind and even body.
> Laughter is a social gesture . . . It pursues a utilitarian aim of general improvement . . . rigidity is comic and laughter is its corrective (Bergson, 1911).

Much of the laughter in class is generated during the movement responses to the question, "How does it feel?" At other times laughter evolves from the movement itself. When we rock forward and backward with our feet swinging up to the ceiling, everybody relaxes, has fun, and laughs. Laughter is an essential ingredient in harmonious group dynamics.

Group Dynamics

Group dynamics is one of the motivational processes. Its ability to stimulate new sources of physical energy and to instill a desire to be part of the body movement group has been discussed in Chapter 9.

A teacher can hasten the feeling of pride in a well-functioning group by systematically inviting individual students to observe

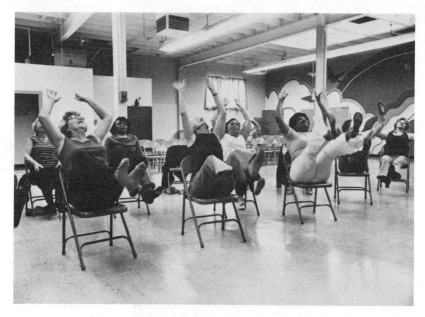

Figure 24. Everyone has fun

one of the larger rhythmic studies from the front of the room. The spectacle of the whole group swinging arms and legs in unison, or rocking from side to side, is truly inspiring. The student observer reacts with pleasure and pride and usually resumes the exercises with greater enthusiasm.

Summary

Since movement itself is nonverbal it must become evident that the most meaningful communication is also achieved non-verbally. Movement is the medium and "the medium is the message."

Verbal communication is auxiliary to the movement. It cues the movement, explains it, and is the social tool for the exchange of ideas. An adequate teacher uses both forms of communication; an inspiring teacher masters them.

12

Improving Posture and Motor Skill

THE EXERCISE MANUAL develops a program to give the body the mobility and strength needed for moderate daily functional movement. This program also reinforces adequate posture—in sitting, standing, walking, and resting. We call this a healthy *postural set*.

The Postural Set

But the term *set* can be misleading, because posture is not a static position. It is an action. Poor posture is a harmful action; it crowds the organs and increases friction in the joints. Good posture is a beneficial action which increases the internal space and is basic to proper body mechanics. Certainly the conscious minute of good posture is as important as any other minute of focused constructive muscular awareness.

To illustrate the benefits of a minute of constructive muscular awareness relative to postural set, focus your students' attention on the neck/head/eye syndrome which is partly responsible for the bent-over posture symptomatic of the aged. The chin tilts up, the eyelids lower, the eyes look down, and the back of the neck shortens. Your students can become aware of these harmful effects in the following exercises:

During a quiet moment of restful exercise, start with eye movements. The students, beginning in Basic Position (see the *Exercise Manual,* Fig. 11), look up and down several times and then continue to look up and down with lids closed. They feel the pulls in the eyes as they change direction and end with the eyes looking straight forward. Follow this exercise with eyelid

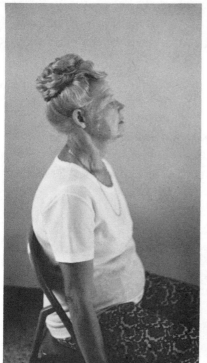 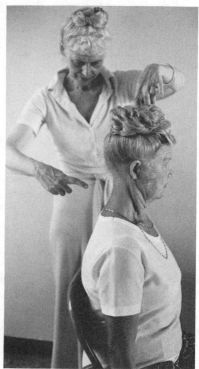

Figure 25. Neck/head/eye syndrome

Figure 26. Correct neck/head/eye pattern

exercises. Squint the eyelids, open them wide, lower, then lift them. Feel the difference in the weight and pull of the lids. Notice the improvement in the view with the lids lifted. Once your students have enjoyed the open eyelids and forward glance of the eyes, you can change the focus and emphasize the stretch of the back of the neck as students push their spines up to the center of the head into Basic Position. Through these simple exercises they build the primary feelings necessary for the correct neck/head/eye relationship.

Now they are ready to recognize this neck/head/eye syndrome in themselves. During a moment when most of the class is relaxed, ask them to freeze, i.e., become immobile. Then follow with these instructions:

1. Maintain your position and become aware of your eyelids. Are they wide open, or are they lowered?
2. Become aware of the back of your neck. Is it shortened or lengthened?
3. Now slowly push your spine up to the top of your head as you push into Basic Position.

After this experience has been repeated several times, the teacher suggests that it is even more helpful to observe another person make these same changes. The teacher may ask for volunteers or may choose a person who likes special attention. It then becomes a sort of game. At any time during the class, ask this person to "freeze." Ask the class to observe this person who now has a clearly visible neck/head/eye syndrome. (The teacher must be confident that the student who has been chosen as the subject does not mind being singled out.) The subject then becomes the model for demonstrating the changing relationship through the same exercise, i.e., maintaining the position and checking the eyelids, becoming aware of the back of the neck, then correcting the syndrome by changing to the correct neck/head/eye pattern through the changes in Basic Position.

As everyone watches the subject move into Basic Position, four changes occur: (1) the back of the neck lengthens; (2) the head tilts forward; (3) the eyelids open; and (4) the eye adjusts and looks straight forward. The class will appreciate the improvement.

After observing the neck/head/eye syndrome and its correction in another person, the participants can become aware of this movement pattern more readily in themselves during or outside class, and can correct it through *one minute of muscular awareness* (one conscious minute) by doing the "three pushes" of Basic Position (see the *Exercise Manual*, Table I-B, Exercise 2) and lifting the eyelids.

Is it really this simple? It *is* quite simple to do, but it is more difficult to maintain. However, if students can remember to go into Basic Position several times a day they will benefit from these "conscious minutes" in improved body-awareness and physical functioning.

Motor Skill

Skill implies a physical technique to be mastered. Specific coordinations are learned, and patterns of coordination are practiced until they become habit. A skill can be considered acquired when it can be performed with little or no deviation, regardless of the stress of the prevailing conditions.

Much of our daily behavior, our "habits," is made up of hidden skills—hidden because they were learned and became habits in a period we no longer remember.

This is true of our motor habits of balance, standing, walking, turning, running, skipping, climbing, falling, rising, lying down, sitting, pushing, pulling, and lifting. It is true of our habits of hygiene as well: bathing, sleeping, dental, and other sanitary practices. Many physical losses attributed to aging are the result of discontinued practice and the eventual breakdown of these hidden skills. This is particularly true of the lack of physical movement with its consequent loss of the flexibility and muscle tone so essential to physical safety during one's normal activity.

It is for this reason that the most pervasively developed skill in our classes is *muscular innervation,* the basis of all movement and movement awareness. As students develop this sensation and get in touch with their physical feelings, they cease to move as if their bodies were a necessary burden and begin to sense movement as a relief and a pleasant experience in itself.

This attitudinal change has a tendency to make one receptive to body-oriented experiences that feel good, such as better posture, increase in daily physical activity, informed relaxation practices, and a feeling of center that improves mental and physical equilibrium. The kinesthetic sense rewards the aware person immediately with the internal confirmation of good feelings. Even a conscious minute of muscular innervation is productive. For the education of any sense is the cumulative effect of repeated practice even if it lasts only a minute at a time.

The cultivation of the kinesthetic sense or any other sense takes time. Look for even slight signs of improvement in your students. Celebrate these improvements with public recognition. Any change in movement awareness is noteworthy. One of the most exciting moments for the Geriatric Body Dynamics teacher, for example, is the sight of a rigid person getting in touch with movement in the lower spine.

Sometimes the improvement that follows the exercise sessions may seem phenomenal, but remember it is not a panacea. Each person can only improve what he or she has. By the age of 65, there may be areas of the body removed or permanently changed by surgery. What we seek in these sessions is improvement, not in the organ itself, but rather in its *functioning*. We cannot exchange used parts for new, but we can add new vigor and better service to what we already have by improving our posture and other motor skills.

Muscular innervation, the basic skill of the kinesthetic sense, then, is critical to our success in helping participants to move and function more effectively. When aging persons can concentrate on the physical sensations of their movement, they can draw the most comfort and pleasure possible from walking, sitting, driving, and other personal and recreational activities.

Simultaneously they can enjoy the physiological benefits of better circulation, respiration, relaxation, and mobility, as well as improved appearance and increased energy for social activities.

We recognize change as the dynamic force in every stage of life and we devote our expertise to influence the changes in senescence toward growth and away from atrophy. Our approach starts with "one conscious minute" of constructive movement. Basic Position is the starting point from which the student continues to develop a heightened sense of body-awareness and movement feelings throughout the Geriatric Body Dynamics Program.

13
Guided Discussion

A WEEKLY hour class in Geriatic Body Dynamics usually includes 15 minutes of discussion. At first, this time may be used for private communication with students, for individual correction and encouragement, or as a question-and-answer period. These moments, set aside from the outset, permit time for the instructor to give special attention to the psychological needs of the individual student while maintaining an uninterrupted flow of movement during the exercise period.

Discussion

After the group has met for several sessions and has begun to feel the unifying influence of group dynamics, a more organized discussion period evolves which is the guided discussion. The purpose of the guided discussion is to motivate continued interest in the movement sessions through (1) involvement, (2) self-expression, and (3) stimulation of self-discoveries and new ideas. It also offers an opportunity to develop more flexible attitudes.

Since this time is set aside from the exercise period, the students may decide whether they wish to participate. They are invited to stay for the discussion after the exercises, and those wishing to leave are given the opportunity to do so gracefully. The remaining students pull their chairs into an intimate circle, while the teacher writes the topic on the chalkboard.

Ideas for discussion take seed at the opening meeting when the students introduce themselves and express their expectations of the program. These expectations become some of the topics.

Often, the students seem reticent initially and have to be encouraged to speak. After a few people participate and the group proves itself to be a safe place psychologically, the more reserved people join in. And as larger numbers of people become more vocal, an informal structure ensures a safe and orderly exchange of ideas.

The teacher, who becomes the facilitator, introduces the ground rules for the guided discussion. The facilitator announces that cross-discussion and conflict of opinion are to be avoided, since this period is an opportunity to express one's thoughts and feelings and not a time to refute the ideas of others. Speakers are urged to be brief so that all who wish to speak may have a chance to do so.

When several people seem eager to talk at once, the facilitator recognizes each one in turn. This is done as informally as possible. Eye contact or a nod of the head often suffices to keep the sequence orderly.

The responses of participants inevitably reflect the kind of facility in which the class is held. Community centers of all kinds host activities for healthier men and women who want to improve their health and appearance. The problems most often expressed here are arthritis, tension, overweight, nutrition, and loneliness.

Residents in retirement homes, by contrast, are more concerned with their own faculties such as sight, hearing, equilibrium, and memory. Touch is a particularly important subject with this group.

Convalescent hospitals and sanitaria present special problems.

Due to the widespread use of tranquilizers and other medication, and the resulting disorientation, communication has to be very stimulating to generate a response.

Feelings of boredom, depression, and anger are characteristic in many of these patients. This period can be an opportunity to ventilate these feelings through movement-oriented imagery-speech games rather than discussion. Figure 27 illustrates such a combination. The rhythmic punching movements accompanied by the shouts of "Pow!" establish a feeling of power which may be directed against the image of an objectionable situation or person.

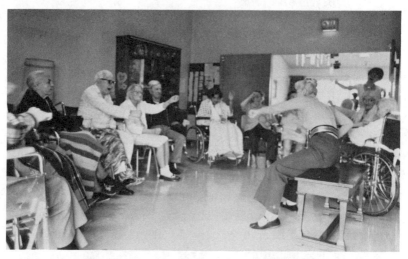

Figure 27. Pow! Hospital patients, several over 90 years old, enjoy the novelty of punching and shouting "Pow!"

The instructor is free to choose from a variety of subjects related to holistic health through body movement. The following five possible discussion areas are listed in relation to class experiences:

1. *Clarification of terms used in class*
   The instructor writes a pair of words on the chalkboard and

allows time for thought. Discussion starts with the question, "Are these two words the same?" Then, using free association, ask, "What ideas pop into your mind with each word?" Write the responses in columns under the related words. The responses listed on the blackboard represent the group thinking. All the ideas are integrated by the facilitator into the concluding presentation of the significance of the two words in relation to movement experience and holistic health.

Discussion arises from such pairs as

 a. *feel* and *sense*
 b. *feel* and *touch*
 c. *look* and *see*
 d. *listen* and *hear*
 e. *sense* and *nonsense*
 f. *senescence* and *senility*
 g. *natural* and *normal*
 h. *balance* and *equilibrium*
 i. *scan* and *read*
 j. *relaxation* and *rest*
 k. *work* and *exercise*
 l. *push* and *pull*

The free association of ideas as a method of expression is equally useful for the other guided discussions for several reasons. It requires a simple, one-word response to participate. Everyone can do it; it is clear; it keeps everyone's attention.

2. *Information for self-improvement*
Discuss the relationship of movement to the biological systems: respiratory system, cardiovascular system, nervous system, and musculo-skeletal system. Discussion of other parts of the body such as skin, ears, eyes, and face also make interesting subjects.

3. *Applications of therapeutic skills*
Scan the body for tension. Dissolve tension through release or relaxation. Relieve leg cramps. Recognize the effects of a

stressful situation on breathing behavior. Increase self-awareness by body-awareness, centering, and grounding techniques.

4. *Development of a holistic viewpoint*
   Discuss the current ideas in the behavioral sciences and arts therapies: holistic health, biofeedback, psychosomatics, touch, imagination, memory, communication, self-image, change, and life-satisfaction. Each category can well be the source of discussion for a whole semester. Many instructors may be more comfortable with their own ideas. The periodicals *The Scientific American* and *Psychology Today* are excellent sources of current information on several of these topics.

The most successful discussions flow directly out of the class experience, and the instructor can plan a lesson (exercises and discussion) around one of the listed topics. For example, if improvement in circulation is the focus of the lesson, then a discussion of the "milking action" of the moving muscles on the veins can be highly motivating. This discussion might be called "A Gift to Your Heart." On the other hand, a student's comment made during the movement session can suggest a practical application of movement to problems such as leg cramps, dizziness, or depression.

Another way to stimulate the students' interest is to write the topic on the blackboard at the beginning of the class. Students see the message and are encouraged to relate it to their thoughts or sensations during the exercises. On the other hand, at times the element of surprise may increase interest when the topic is unexpectedly written at the end of the exercise period.

These written statements require thought and creativity. They are phrased to excite curiosity or the students' sense of humor. All statements are read aloud at the start of the discussion period. If the statement is fanciful or tricky, it sets a light mood. Consider

113

the surprise of the men and women who are asked to read "I am sensational!" (A discussion of sensation and sensory awareness follows.)

A significant aspect of the guided discussion is its influence on flexibility in communication. The participants tend to listen more closely as apparent differences of opinion are woven into unified ideas. This experience also tends to soften opposition to the opinions of others because the discussions demonstrate that someone else's idea need not be wrong for one's own idea to be right. This mental flexibility may be enhanced by such other psychologically oriented subjects as: tension-forming emotions and ideas (worry, anger, stubborness), and their effect on muscles, nerves, and breathing.

Whatever the topic, the instructor always remembers to approach it flexibly, using student interest and participation as one of the guides for judging which direction to take. Having introduced relevant information during discussions, the instructor continues the educational process with a pattern of constructive suggestions. Those students who have trust and confidence in the instructor are particularly responsive to specific suggestions for home practice of relaxation, nutrition, exercise, and a more flexible attitude toward their problems.

The guided discussion period enormously increases the potential for re-evaluation and change. For instance, after discussion of a holistic approach to health, men and women are better prepared to take reponsibility for coping with some of their own psychosomatically-induced symptoms. Let's look at one example of the results of discussions on this subject:

Dorothy, who has high blood pressure, always got a "sick headache" when her husband turned the television to football, baseball, or hockey games. She took two aspirin and tried to go to sleep, as she silently blamed him for her condition.

Now Dorothy has re-evaluated the situation. She leaves the living room before the television sports programs begin. She takes the opportunity to practice relaxation exercises for a few minutes and then feels good enough to enjoy one of her hobbies during the rest of the evening. Dorothy's attitude has become more flexible. She has changed her own behavior to correct her headache.

14
The Lecture Demonstration

AMONG THE MANY rewarding experiences possible in an advanced group is a class demonstration. The movement ritual is visually dynamic; the concentration, use of rhythm, and unison movement of a Geriatric Body Dynamics class lend themselves to a performance. The students are proud of their personal and group achievement and are enthusiastic about sharing this valuable experience with their peers.

Therefore, a well-functioning class needs little, if any, additional preparation. If the demonstration is to be held in a different room, it helps to rehearse the entrance and exit to and from the new place.

Are there possible problems? Since a demonstration implies an audience, we are faced with the same problems that a nonparticipating guest presents in a regular class. Therefore, the instructor precedes every demonstration with a brief orientation which includes audience participation. The audience is then invited to participate during the class demonstration as well.

Here is an example of how the orientation to a lecture demonstration might start (the class is seated on chairs on the stage; the teacher is downstage, in front of them facing the audience):

Welcome to you all, and thank you for joining us today. If I say the word *exercise*, you retired men and women in the audience may think, "Sure, exercise is good for somebody else. I'm lucky if I can get up out of my chair and take a walk!" But suppose we say "You don't have to get up out of your chair!" You may reply, "Then, what good is it?"

Well the men and women demonstrating will give you the answer.

The exercises which you will see are designed within your limitations. These exercises begin when your breadwinning and homemaking jobs diminish or end. They supplement the physical activity essential to trigger improved circulation, flexibility of the joints, healthier nerves, easier breathing—now—today—and they ward off the dreaded day of increasing dependence on others.

The people you see in this demonstration could easily be you. While you watch Jack, who just celebrated his eighty-eighth birthday; and Betty, who has been attending this class about five years; and Sam, who started with us only a month ago; you can discover the pleasure of these exercises doing them along with us.

How many of you would like to try? Raise your hands. Good! Let's make this our first exercise. Stretch one arm up to the ceiling with me, and let it drop. Stretch the other arm way up, and let it drop. And now let's extend both arms up and stretch first one side and then the other. Open them wide out to the side and down.

And now will the rest of you join us? Let's put our purses under the seats so that we are free to move. Men, won't you unbutton your jackets? Let's sit way back in our chairs. (Teacher is now seated.)

We all move to the same direction—just mirror me. When I lift my arm on this side, you lift your arm on the same side. (If necessary, point to the side near the window or whatever distinguishes that side of the room from the other.) Now change and lean to the other side. When I lean forward, you lean forward. That's fine. Lean backward with me. And now we are ready to start.

The teacher may continue to lead the audience as she starts the demonstration, or s/he may face the group on the stage and encourage the audience to follow them. If the teacher chooses to face the audience, the demonstration group will mirror the teacher's back. Therefore their movements will start on their left side, just as the teacher's movement does. If she faces the demonstration group, the audience, now mirroring the teacher's back, will start to their left.

The teacher has to evaluate the situation. If the majority of the audience is ready to participate, then audience participation takes priority. If the audience is not ready to join in as a group, the demonstration becomes the motivator and the teacher faces the class as usual to stimulate their confidence, enthusiasm, and skill for an inspiring performance.

There is one more possibility that has to be considered: is the teacher experienced enough to lead the demonstration and the participation? If there is any doubt, the teacher will do well to conduct several demonstrations before encouraging audience participation.

A demonstration is a performance and as such has to have visual interest, good timing, and an interesting subject. For visual interest the group performs on a platform. All the women wear slacks. Encourage the use of bright color in shirts or scarfs. And, of course, the exercises themselves and the arrangement of the order they follow must be timed to maintain attention and interest.

The subject of the demonstration, chair exercises, is unique. It is interesting both because it is unusual and because it is the solution to the problem of exercise for all people who cannot participate for physical reasons in regular fitness, sports, or dance activities.

For the substance of the demonstration, the exercise studies, the teacher has the model of the instructional cassette, *Invitation To Exercise*. It is material that can be mounted on the stage as it is. Some teachers may find one of the other cassettes more appropriate. The more experienced teacher has a greater number of choices.

The accompaniment the teacher chooses depends on the resources available. The occasional use of singing voices in self-accompaniment is interesting, appropriate, and the least complicated. The rhythmic effect of castanets used by the teacher can perk up the audience and emphasize the unison and accent of the movements. A teacher who normally uses taped music or records to accompany the movement during class will be able to use them effectively during the demonstration. The class which has been fortunate enough to have a live accompanist during class will, of course, have the accompanist for the demonstration.

The conclusion of a performance is very important. It carries the message of the purpose of the demonstration. The purpose of these chair exercises is to stimulate, exhilarate, and infuse each person with the joy of moving.

The teacher who uses the *Invitation to Exercise* sequences may use the forward and backward rocking to build momentum, and rocking forward with the weight on the feet a few times (still within the pattern of the rocking motion) and finishing with the weight on the feet and standing. The final swing upwards brings the person upright with both hands in the air.

Another rousing conclusion can be achieved with a side-to-side rocking and singing movement. The people extend both arms out to the side and around the shoulders of the persons next to them. They start rocking to the same side and the teacher suggests a song that most of them know, e.g., "When the Saints Go Marching In" or some other equally stimulating melody. The words are unimportant. Just "la la la" the tune and at the end, finish on a high note. This may mean singing the last note an octave higher than written.

The demonstration is over. Most of the people are laughing and talking. What, if any, are the more lasting results of this entertaining presentation of a class lesson? You may expect to discover (1) increased group spirit of the performing class, (2) appreciation and acknowledgment of the students' achievements by the audience, (3) better public relations for the program, (4) the establishment of Geriatric Body Dynamics as an important, attractive, and desirable senior adult activity in your community, and (5) people in the audience will want to join the class.

15
Starting a Geriatric Body Dynamics Class

IT IS TIME to raise some of the practical questions of starting a Geriatric Body Dynamics class.

Publicity

The men and women who *need* this activity have to hear about it before they can join it. They have to know where and when a class is available. To assure that such announcements are received, you will want to consider both publicity and public relations.

Advance publicity should reach two main groups. These are (1) those people whom you wish to involve in the class, and (2) the personnel of the facility that houses the activity, particularly the employees who have direct contact with your potential students.

Some illustrations of kinds of publicity and other suggestions follow. You may use these as a model or as a springboard for your own ideas. Every group is different, and the uniqueness of each group should be recognized not only in the publicity but in all the other aspects of the Geriatric Body Dynamics class.

YOUR HEALTH I.Q.

	True	False
1. People over 80 should sit more.	___	___
2. The more sleep you get, the more energy you have.	___	___
3. Cleaning your room and exercise classes give the same results.	___	___
4. The more you rest, the better it is for your heart.	___	___
5. Everybody breathes naturally.	___	___
6. Good exercise is strenuous.	___	___
7. Only drugs can improve circulation.	___	___
8. The only way to keep your bones strong is by diet.	___	___
9. Blinking is a sign of weakness.	___	___
10. Relaxation and rest are synonymous.	___	___

FOR ANSWERS TO THESE QUESTIONS,
TURN THIS PAGE UPSIDE DOWN.

The answer to all ten questions is *False.* If you want to discuss these questions, come to our Geriatric Body Dynamics class on _____ at _____ in _____.

Figure 28.   A Health I.Q. Quiz designed to interest senior adults in movement classes

Starting a Geriatric Body Dynamics Class

You can stimulate interest before the first class through

1. Newspaper releases
2. Announcements in news bulletins
3. Quizzes
4. Bulletin board announcements
5. Announcements during meal times (in retirement or nursing homes)
6. Preregistration

A quiz might be developed along the lines shown in Figure 28. A copy of this quiz was placed in each resident's mail box in one retirement home. It was published in the monthly news bulletin of another home and posted on a bulletin board of still another. It stimulated conversations at the dining table and served as an excellent introduction to the opening lesson of the Geriatric Body Dynamics class.

Ideas for an article (for which you can include pictures) are suggested by the following story, reprinted from the *National Benevolent Association News Bulletin.*

EXERCISE FOR OPTIMAL AGING*

"I LOVE IT!" It is stimulating and relaxing at the same time. I feel so very much better after I participate. "Try it, you'll like it," says Mrs. Jacks, 78-year-old member of the "Exercise for Optimal Aging" class.

COME RAIN OR SHINE, every Thursday morning 25 residents of the California Christian Home gather for chair exercises and discussion relevant to their physical and mental health.

THIS CLASS IS TAUGHT by Eva Desca Garnet, M.S., as part of the Adult Education Extension Program of Mr. Richard Manning, principal of the Mountain View School. Mr. Jack Billingsley, Administrator of the Home, says that all of the participating residents are between the ages of 71 and 91. Among the several activities provided to the residents, Mr. Billingsley insists on the exercise being a top priority for all those who can participate.

THE REASON FOR THEIR FAITHFUL ATTENDANCE soon becomes

*This is the name given to the Geriatric Body Dynamics Class at this retirement home.

clear as their sighs change from *Ouch* to *Ahhhh,* expressing their relief from tight painful muscles. As the class progresses, smiles and laughter punctuate the enjoyment of these therapeutic as well as educational and recreational experiences.

DURING ONE OF THE DISCUSSIONS on the value of the exercise, paticipant Dr. John Long, retired English professor, commented:

"The laws of nature illustrate in many ways that what we don't use, we lose. This is certainly true of our own bodies. No matter what our age, we need continued exercise. Our class has demonstrated so beautifully the ways that people of even the most limited physical ability can experience and improve themselves."

THROUGH THE MANY OPPORTUNITIES for new learning experiences the mind is stimulated as well. Mrs. Stole, another member of the class, expressed it this way:

"What's so important are the talks on the function of the body as one organ relates to another: like the red blood corpuscles relate to respiration and circulation and the effect of exercise on muscles and bones. I think this is as important as exercise because it explains what the movements mean to our bodies. Then we want to do these exercises to get these excellent results.

I enjoy this aspect immensely. I was an enthusiastic physiology student and this stimulates my past interest in this exciting study."

NOR ARE THE EMOTIONS NEGLECTED. A whole range of pleasant feelings are also stimulated through the use of imagination and heightened awareness, particularly in the muscles. This sense is known as the "kinesthetic sense" and can be very useful therapeutically. Members have learned to apply it in dealing with leg cramps as well as other minor discomforts. They say it helps them reduce tension headaches, neck and shoulder pains, discomfort from gas, and stiffness in the joints.

SUCH EXPERIENCES AFFECT THE WAY elderly people feel about themselves and their lives. "Exercise for Optimal Aging" helps increase the satisfaction these men and women feel with themselves. This improved outlook helps them meet the people they live with in a happier frame of mind.

Starting a Geriatric Body Dynamics Class

The staff is crucial to the success of any activity, especially in a retirement home, nursing home, or hospital. The therapist gets the best results where s/he can address an orientation session attended by the activity director, nurses, and aides before the first class meeting. Such a lecture stresses the benefits the staff as well as the residents derive from this activity.

At such a briefing the therapist's remarks are aimed at the enlightened self-interest of the staff. The staff is generally overworked by the large number of patients they care for, and overstressed by the endless calls for personal attention. Reliable information that can lighten the work load or lessen the stress will command attention and generate cooperation.

The staff and administration can relate to the quotation from the *Sanitaria Magazine* that follows:

> The direct benefits of Geriatric-Calisthenics* classes have been stated by administrators who have seen these results:
> "It provides a better patient atmosphere; it provides an important form of group activity and interaction. At a certain level of recovery it provides a positive physiological activity which enables the patient to better handle himself and minimize complaints.
> "It improves patient control. By providing a constructive use of energy, it results in relaxation and gentle fatigue that offsets typical manifestations of frustration and hostility which are part of the management problems.
> "A Geriatric-Calisthenics class is dramatic evidence to families of patients that more than custodial care is offered their loved ones. It provides a service that requires very little capital investment."

If time permits, the therapist can introduce scientific evidence of the relationship between inactivity, boredom, and mental disorientation. Especially appropriate is the information on experimental sensory deprivation described in "The Pathology of Boredom." Woodburn Heron, experimental psychologist, writes,

*Another name for G. B. D.

"Monotony is an important and enduring problem." Sensory deprivation causes the brain to behave abnormally. His laboratory experiments are confirmed by examples from real life situations:

"Studies in France and Harvard University ... (reveal that) hallucinations (are) common among long distance truck drivers ... apparitions such as giant red spiders on the windshield (and) non-existent animals crossing the road. Similarly (affected are) aviators on long flights ... Charles A. Lindberg described some in his autobiography." Heron comes to the conclusion, "Variety is not the spice of life, it is the very stuff of it" (1957).

Parallels between experimental conditions of sensory deprivation and the living conditions of long-term patients are inescapable, particularly as most elderly patients suffer partial sensory deprivation due to impairment of sight and hearing, and minimal stimulation of touch and movement. The therapist can suggest the relevance of the sensory stimulation aspects of the Body Dynamics Program to a reality-orientation program.

Stimulating the senses is the biological approach to reality. It puts people in touch with themselves, their partners, and their environment.

At the conclusion of the orientation session, the instructor may ask for a staff person to serve as liaison between the instructor and the residents, and for an interested resident to act as the group's secretary. The instructor later meets the staff liaison, discusses questions, and offers the quiz or any other handout that has to be reproduced. The secretary distributes them, speaks to residents, and gets a list of people who plan to attend.

The instructor can contribute articles to the monthly newsletter or bulletin mimeographed by the staff. One article can report on the people who plan to participate in the class. Another article, perhaps written by a staff member, might report on the instructor, his or her credentials, and the popularity of both the instructor and the program at other institutions.

Starting a Geriatric Body Dynamics Class

Older people need constant reminders. An attractive poster, similar to Figure 29, announces the class a week before it starts. On the day the class meets, an announcement appears on the daily schedule of the bulletin board:

Health and Movement Class—10:00 A.M.—Chapel

or whatever seems appropriate. Especially important is an announcement made at breakfast, reminding the people who have registered to attend. The announcer can open the door to future participants by inviting everyone else to come and meet the teacher too. As a final cue, some activity directors ring a hand bell in the corridors to alert residents that an activity is about to start.

JOIN OUR HEALTH AND MOVEMENT CLASS

BODY DYNAMICS

Monday Mornings

When: _____

Where: _____

Meet the Teacher, _____ (insert name) _____

For more information speak to _____

_____

Figure 29. "Advance poster." Announcement of Geriatric Body Dynamics class

125

Community centers and other public places have their own preregistration procedures. They make more extensive use of local newspapers, posters, and announcements at other club meetings and activities. Sometimes they have radio publicity in the form of a Calendar of Events as a public service. Discuss all these possibilities with the publicity director and the staff person in charge of senior citizens' activities.

For newspaper publicity, submit a glossy photograph of yourself, a typed autobiographical sketch, and the announcement of the class time, place, and purpose, as well as a copy of the quiz. There is no way of knowing in advance what material will actually be printed.

Because most community centers have a formal preregistration, a list of the prospective students may be available to you. This list can help you to become familiar with your students' names before you meet them.

How Long, How Large, How Often?

Where an activity director or therapist is employed on the staff of a residential home or sanatorium, daily exercise activity is desirable. This can be an exercise break from another activity such as Bingo or Arts and Crafts or during music sessions as well as a scheduled Geriatric Body Dynamics class. For actual exercise sessions, the class size may be increased above fifteen in convalescent hospitals where aides are available. A nurse or aide may also run an evening session in relaxation to promote sleep. Facial and eye exercises are especially relaxing in such evening programs.

Up to 20 men and women can join a class in all other facilities, including special senior adult centers, nutrition centers, union halls, churches and temples, small board and care homes, hotels, golden age clubs, and community centers. As many classes as are feasible should be planned. Even a group that meets but once a month benefits from the experience.

Starting a Geriatric Body Dynamics Class

The class lasts one hour. Once it starts, it continues without interruptions of any kind. Explanations are made during the movements. As described in Chapter 13, the last 15 minutes of the class may be used for discussion.

Daily schedules may include hours in the morning, afternoon, and evening. A class should start 1 to 1½ hours after a light meal, 2 to 2½ hours after a heavy meal. This usually makes available:

MORNINGS:	9:30 to 12:00 noon
AFTERNOONS:	2:30 to 5:00 P.M.
EVENINGS:	7:00 to 8:30 P.M.

Where Geriatric Body Dynamics is one of many physical fitness activities, a student may enjoy participating for one semester and change to another activity for the next semester. But where it is the only physical activity possible for the student, it may become and continue to be as regular as any other habit.

Is there advancement for the student who has improved? Where graded classes are possible, there can be three levels of participation: fundamental, intermediate, and advanced. The degree of improvement varies with the student's physical condition and ability to concentrate. Because students have their own individual limitations, they may be working at the highest and deepest levels of their capacity and yet comfortably remain in a fundamental class.

Therefore, we do not think in terms of automatic advancement. Rather, we consider the intermediate and advanced classes as opportunities for those in better health to enrich their physical experience.

The student in an intermediate class has mastered rhythmic breathing, Basic Position Forward, swings, "reading" movement, and concentration. A person in this class has the physical capacity to stand up and sit down *without* any physical assistance.

127

Students in an advanced class, in addition to the requirements for an intermediate class, have developed awareness of innervation, relaxation, coordination, and muscular vitality; and they can walk with comfort.

Where conditions permit more than one class, the instructor can set up graded classes. There are groups that continue to meet once a week for years. These participants may be ready for the complex coordinations of the intermediate or advanced classes even though some may have difficulty standing or walking. In such a class, the handicapped students participate when they can and enjoy the psychomotor challenge of keeping pace with the level of the class.

Ideal Room Setting

The ritual of the class starts with the room setting. The activity should be scheduled in a spacious, calm, and beautiful room. It may be a studio, chapel, activity room, or TV room, and often requires the moving of furniture to clear space for the set-up. The ideal arrangement includes twelve to fifteen folding chairs, one for each member of the class, and a table for personal belongings of the students. A low platform is set up for the teacher. A folding chair with a microphone (lavaliere or standing mike) is stationed in the middle of the platform. An electric cord, cassette tape recorder, or record player are placed at the right side, and flowers or a plant perk up the left side. A blackboard rises behind the platform.

The chairs are arranged in a gentle curve, about two or three feet apart. The instructor's chair (in the center of the platform) faces the curve of students' chairs, about eight feet in front of the class. An alternative arrangement of two concentric curves with the chairs two or three feet apart may be used. Chairs in the back curve are set in the spaces between the front chairs. The second plan works well when the room is small or some of the students are shy.

This "arc" seating arrangement focuses attention on the teacher, making the student less likely to focus on his or her neighbors and be irritated or influenced by their performance. Each student is provided enough space to move freely in the chair, without interference. All the students can see the teacher, see the demonstrated movements, and hear the constant verbal instruction without strain. After the second meeting, the students generally have (and feel at home in) their own seats.

The classroom may have doors to shut out distracting sounds and ensure privacy. A comfortable 72 degree Fahrenheit (25° C) temperature is desirable. The room should be well lighted, but the instructor may wish to avoid sun glare by closing the draperies. There should be fresh air but no draft. The floor should be dry mopped before the class to avoid the students' inhaling dust.

Each student is within easy vision of the teacher so the teacher can rely on eye contact and give individual attention so essential to safety and motivation. The teacher must be able to read simple changes of facial expression, whether it is the pallor of dizziness, flush of exertion, or the relaxed expression and smile of pleasure.

This physical arrangement of the room gives structure to the ritual and substance to the context of individual attention and recognition within the form of group activity.

Figure 30 illustrates an ideal arrangement. Any (or many) of the items listed may not be available. The instructor who is aware of the need each item serves, however, will compensate for its lack in some way.

Each article of equipment serves a therapeutic purpose. The platform improves visibility and eye contact. Its one- or two-foot height makes the instructor's movements visible to all the sighted people in the room. The instructor can see the total form of the seated students and can make eye contact with each one. The microphone makes the instructor's voice more audible, especially for the unsighted and weak-sighted students who rely solely on the voice, and for the partially deaf. It also improves reception for people with hearing aids.

The flowers or plant on the instructor's left orients the students to direction. The side movements always start in the direction of the flowers; they provide an additional cue for those students who don't respond immediately to the "mirror me" technique. Flowers or a plant also introduce an aesthetic aspect.

A good metal folding chair with a leather pad has many advantages. Such a chair is strong, stable, generally well-proportioned for depth of the seat and height from the floor, and has the proper pitch for support to the back. The chair permits freedom for movements such as rocking while ensuring solid, stable support. Yet it is light enough to move into other seating arrangements, as in pairing. The leather pad ensures warm, comfortable contact. And, finally, such chairs are easily stacked so that the room can be set up quickly and the chairs can be removed swiftly in preparation for the next activity.

The floor plan in Figure 30 is used for ambulatory men and women. As discussed above, they sit in concentric curves facing the teacher, who is seated on a platform. During seated pairing exercises, the participants can turn their chairs to face another person at the side or in back of them. People who use walkers and can sit in straight-backed chairs also fit into this setup.

The floor plan in Figure 31 is used for wheelchairs. It shows an oval pattern of wheelchairs, with some folding chairs interspersed for patients who can be transferred into them with the help of aides. The participants seated in the "circle" are within hands' distance of each other. This arrangement does not use the platform for improved sight lines and requires the activity director and/or aides for increased contact and manual instruction. (When patients have visitors, invite them to join in and help with the class.)

In this pattern, the leader has a chair in the circle, as do the aides, strategically placed for partnering people who are espe-

Starting a Geriatric Body Dynamics Class

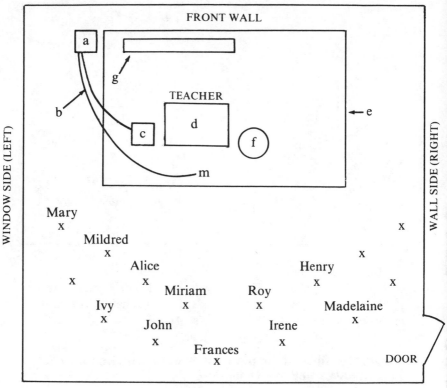

a   Electrical wall outlet   f   Flowers or plant
b   Electrical cords   g   Blackboard
    (Extension cord,   m   Microphone
    if necessary)   x's   Folding chairs for students
c   Cassette recorder
d   Teacher's chair
e   Platform

Figure 30. Ideal floor plan for a class. The walls are labeled from the students' point of view. A chart of the chair arrangement with the name of each student written above each X, as illustrated, aids the instructor in recalling students' names

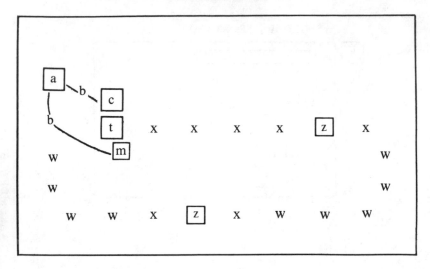

a	Electrical outlet
b	Electrical cord
c	Casette recorder
m	Microphone

t	Teacher
w's	Wheelchair participants
x's	Folding chair participants
z's	Aides

Figure 31. Ideal floor plan for a class with some or all participants using wheelchairs

cially handicapped. The leader and aides also move around to other patients, as needed, and return to home base.

The microphone and tape recorder are arranged conveniently by the leader's chair. The location of the electrical outlet generally determines where the leader will sit. Even though the placement of wheelchair patients is more difficult to control, the instructor tries to place them in the same areas with the same partners for every class meeting.

Two other seating arrangements will be used during the class. We touched on the first, *pairing,* in discussing Figure 30. In wheelchairs, pairing is done in a loveseat position. The partners face each other with their chairs overlapping so that their right sides are adjacent as in Figure 32.

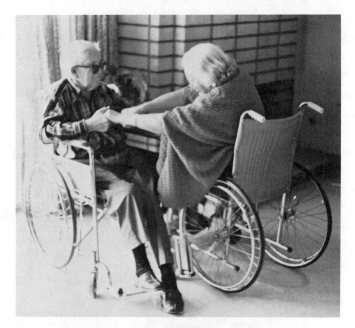

Figure 32. Loveseat arrangement

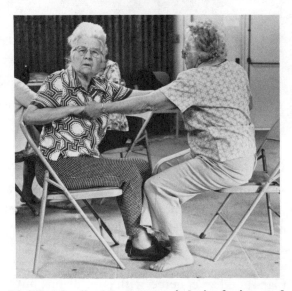

Figure 33. "Pairing" with partners' chairs facing each other

In cases where the patient's right side is handicapped, the wheelchairs are arranged so that the partners' left sides are adjacent. Pairing is simpler, of course, with regular chairs; the two partners' chairs are turned to face each other.

We term the second special seating arrangement *chair squares*, used with the tape cassettes *Rhythm and Rhyme in Country Dance Time* and *Chair Skwairs*. Here a square is formed by four sets of partners (eight chairs, two on each side) facing the center. The sets are arranged closely enough so that the participants may hold hands to form a circle without strain.

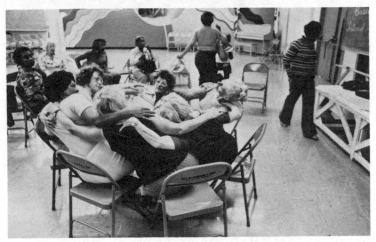

Figure 34. Chair squares used for adaptation of square dancing

Clothing

"Clothes have a very important mental effect on the person ... accessories of different colors do give emotional variety ..." (Lawton, p. 199). The teacher and students dress appropriately for exercise. The clothing should be comfortable, flexible, and attractive. Since slacks are most appropriate for leg movements, men have no problem. In *hospitals,* many of the men and women have their laps and legs covered with comforters, but these don't seem to restrict their movements. In other settings, appropriate

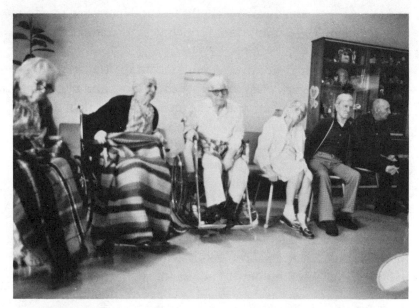

Figure 35. Many men and women cover their laps with comforters

dress for the women is often determined by the state of their health, the rules of the institution, and the sense of propriety of the participants. Fortunately, many older women now wear slacks.

A problem arises in institutions, however, when rules do not permit women to wear pants outfits in the dining room. In such cases, changing clothing is often a more difficult chore than it appears to be. A clothing change may involve a long trip to one's room—changing out of pants and into a dress, foundation garments, and stockings; and it may also involve the re-dressing of hair.

Where pants suits are practical, women are encouraged to wear them. They may wear wide-skirted dresses or skirts if slacks are not practical.

If possible, ask your students to wear cotton socks. Cotton socks relieve the feet of the restriction of the tight fit of stockings

135

and allow for greater awareness in the feet and increased freedom of movement. This is important for people with diabetes or poor circulation.

Where warmth is not a problem, encourage the students at some point during the class to remove their shoes and place them under their seats. Similarly, urge the men to remove their jackets. Usually the shedding of sweaters occurs as the exercise proceeds.

The instructor's verbal recognition of appropriate dress, bright colors, cotton socks, and the removal of shoes reinforces the students' desire to dress appropriately for each exercise session.

The teacher's image is part of the ritual. Many people attend because of the lift in spirit they experience when they see the teacher. The color and fabric of the outfit are partly responsible for this effect. The teacher projects a well-groomed look, entering the class in a teaching outfit chosen for:

1. Appropriateness for movement.
2. Appropriateness for the teacher's personality.
3. Appropriateness for the students.

The teacher's clothing should be flexible and reveal the body movements. A leotard or a knitted or jersey top, for example, could be complemented by a pair of matching or color-coordinated pants.

The color of the teacher's clothing is important to the success of the instruction. Bright color is seen more easily and stimulates the eye and the attention in general. Color also has emotional significance and must be used judiciously. White is cool. Blue is calming; purple, warm; pink and gold, cheerful; red, exciting; pastels, relaxing. Weather and student mood should also guide choice in color. Wear cool colors in warm weather and cheerful colors for hospitals.

Students' comments on the teacher's clothing are considered a key to their approval and to the degree it stimulates them. The choice of colors and designs may be modified by the needs of the students, including their handicaps (vision), prejudice (tights), and preferences (color).

A teacher should have at least two outfits of different colors and alternate them as needed. Clothes should reflect body-image and the body as an instrument rather than the competitiveness of athletics as would be suggested, for example, by a jogging suit. In short, the teacher's clothes should establish an aesthetic, flexible, vital appearance that is the keynote of the whole movement ritual.

Introductory Part of the First Class

These considerations may seem endless to a new instructor, even though they quickly become second nature—almost a simple matter of "common sense." The following checklist can help both new and seasoned instructors be certain the initial class goes smoothly:

1. Set up the room before the students enter.
2. Greet each student as s/he enters the room, shaking hands and connecting name and person physically. Take attendance. Ask each person if there is something special about his or her health that you should know. Assign seats based on student preference. (Often students will choose seats for the first session, and you need only request that they keep the same seats for future meetings.)
3. Check on safety and comfort:
   a. Light—correct too much glare or too little light by adjusting draperies, changing the angle of light bulbs, or getting more light.
   b. Temperature—check windows, heater, or air conditioner.

c. Sight lines—can everyone see you? Can you see everyone?
d. Noise—where possible, reduce the noise level.
e. Chairs—are they steady and sturdy?

When everyone is settled in chairs and comfortable, move on to your own procedure, perhaps based on the following suggestions:

Introduce yourself officially and introduce the secretary, if one has been appointed (as suggested on page 124). Thank the people who helped to make the event possible. Ask for a show of hands of people who are registered if this is appropriate. Greet all visitors, and open the class with a question: "What would you like to get from this class?" Write the responses on the blackboard.

Address yourself to the participants' comments. Relate the rest of your introduction to their desires as expressed and listed on the blackboard. Suggest that future activity and discussions will be based on these interests. Lead naturally into the concept, "The body—the instrument," and start the exercises with Tape I, Side A of *Invitation to Exercise.*

Groups in convalescent hospitals may continue to use Side A for several sessions and their movement experience may be expanded with the introduction of appropriate "studies" from some of the other cassettes.

All other groups may go immediately from the movements of Side A to Side B in the first class lesson. Tape I, Side B is the basic exercise lesson. All of the other tapes are developments of the movement ideas and "studies" presented in *Invitation to Exercise.*

Instructional Tapes

The instructional tapes that accompany this text are models of the Geriatric Body Dynamics approach. They are practical applications of its theory and principles. In-depth study of these tapes is facilitated through the use of the tapescripts and photographs presented in the *Exercise Manual.*

Best results can be achieved through a whole-part-whole pattern of learning. This conforms with the Gestalt Psychology principle that we naturally apprehend events as a whole and then, as we analyze them, the individual parts are more meaningful because they retain a significant relationship to the total event. When we return to the whole experience again it has become enriched by the deeper understanding of its elements.

This is accomplished by hearing the whole exercise tape and actually following the instructions without interruption. After getting the sense of the whole lesson, combine the playing of the tape with the reading of the text, study the tapescript and the illustrations as they implement the oral instructions. By hearing the instructions, subvocalizing the tapescript, and seeing the photographic illustrations, the teacher gets a multisensory experience of the movement.

After several repetitions of this process, the teacher begins to experience the feelings, the shape, the tempo, the value, and the relationship of the sequences of the movement as a whole experience. Simultaneously s/he internalizes the verbal flow of instructions. The whole-part-whole pattern is used in teaching as well. Each unit of study (see the *Exercise Manual*) starts with an instructional tape and the subsequent lesson plans emphasize successive exercises by giving extra time and attention to understanding and experiencing each exercise more fully.

This process of learning involves both the right and left hemispheres of the brain as well as total involvement of the mind and body. The person who learns the approach holistically is better prepared to teach it holistically.

Geriatric Body Dynamics is always concerned with the whole person. As the students move along the health continuum toward well-being and exhilaration, and as they improve physically and demonstrate greater movement-readiness, the scope of movement possibilities grows with them.

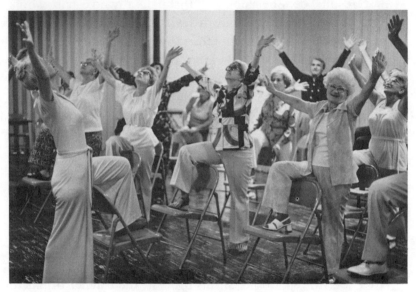

Figure 36. As movement-readiness grows, movement possibilities grow

Conclusion

As the gap is bridged between the process of aging and vital living, preparation for retirement is becoming more important to middle-age adults. This is particularly true of their growing interest in body-awareness and exercise. People in their middle forties and early fifties are flocking to movement activities as a form of health insurance and recreation.

The number of people who continue with these activities after they retire is also increasing. As a result, there is emerging a new dynamic image of the older adult. This is both a gratifying change and a stimulating challenge.

Many of these men and women are younger physically and psychologically if not biologically. Body movement must be geared to the increased physical tolerance of this group but their health must not be taken for granted. Check their disabilities; check their pulse rates.

Therapists must maintain and improve their own health holistically and continue to be a model for this new, vital older generation.

16

The Moment of Truth

SOON YOU WILL teach your first class—if you have not already done so. Picture yourself at that "moment of truth" now. Maybe it's in a convalescent hospital, a retirement home, or a senior citizen center. You have prepared yourself for this important event with considerable care. Nevertheless, you are probably feeling a rising anxiety as several questions keep repeating in your mind. You are asking yourself, "How should I start? What should I do? How will I keep them interested?" In reviewing these questions, you see that each one begins with the word, "I." So, let's start with that.

How do you really feel about teaching a class of body movement to aging people? There are actually five parts to this query:

1. First, ask yourself how you feel about body movement. Do you enjoy the physical sensation of expressing energy through your body, or do you express your vitality through your voice instead?
2. Then ask yourself how you feel about teaching. Do you feel the exhilaration of sharing a precious

experience and enjoy stimulating others to discover this experience for themselves? Or is it a job that you dutifully perform to the best of your ability?

3. How do you feel about teaching body movement? Do you participate and teach vitalizing exercises by example? Or do you expect your students to "do as you say, not as you do?"

4. Can you lead a class emphasizing the body-image with confidence? Or would you rather retreat under the anonymity of loose clothes and hide the very instrument you are teaching your students to discover?

5. How do you think older people value exercise? Do they believe it is useless to make an effort? Or can you anticipate this class as an opportunity to stimulate people's faith in themselves and in their own improvement?

The answers to these questions reveal how well-prepared you are to answer the final question: *"How will I keep them interested?"* Assuming that you have answered the previous questions satisfactorily, and assuming that you have the knowledge and skill of teaching Geriatric Body Dynamics (or any other form of adapted exercise for older people), the answer is simple. Be interested in your students.

When you, the teacher, change your conscious awareness from yourself to focus upon the group, an incredible change occurs. It frees the group of its own self-consciousness and promotes an involvement that surpasses interest.

The transformation that every teacher hopes for comes to pass. The students' attitudes change from disinterest or mere curiosity to involvement, and from boredom or even pain, to pleasure. Each person becomes revitalized, freer, and happier as a person and in concert with the community.

When you watch this transformation you will find, as I have, that the rewards of this work in affection, creative energy, and a deepening sense of life for both you and your students is immeasurable. Our field is enriched when the quality of your being is as important to your students as the activity you bring. What you are to these people is a connection to *living*. They empathize with your energy and enthusiasm.

Throughout the writing of this book and preparation of the accompanying tapes and *Exercise Manual,* my purpose has been to bring you confidently to this, your challenging moment.

Bibliography

Adams, David L. "Analysis of Life Satisfaction Index," *Journal of Gerontology,* XXIV:4, October 1969, pp. 470-474.

American Institute of Planners and American Association of Health, Physical Education and Recreation. "Leisure and the Quality of Life," *Survey of Participants in Leisure and the Quality of Life Conference,* Part III, March 8-11, 1970, La Costa, California.

American Medical Association. "Vigorous Exercise at Any Age Even After Infarct Is Upheld," *Medical Tribune,* January 10, 1966.

Anderson, John E. "Background Paper on Research in Gerontology: Psychological and Social Sciences." Prepared under the Planning Committee on Research in Gerontology, Psychology and Social Sciences, April, 1960, for the White House Conference on Aging, 1961.

Anderson, Virgil A. *Training the Speaking Voice.* New York: Oxford University Press, 1961.

Bergson, Henri. *Laughter, An Essay on the Meaning of the Comic.* New York: Macmillan, 1911.

Berne, Eric, M.D. *Transactional Analysis in Psychotherapy.* New York: Grove Press, 1961.

Birren, James E. *Psychology of Aging.* Englewood Cliffs, N.J.: Prentice-Hall, 1964.

Birren, James E. et al. "Research, Demonstration, and Training : Issues and Methodology in Social Gerontology," *The Gerontologist,* Summer 1972, Part II, p. 54.

Birren, Faber. *Color Psychology and Color Therapy.* New Hyde Park, N.Y.: University Books, 1961.

Bloomfield, Harold H., M.D. and Robert B. Kory. *The Holistic Way to Health and Happiness.* New York: Simon and Schuster, 1978.

Bock, George and Yetta Bernhard. *Aggression Lab.* Dubuque, Iowa: Kendall/Hunt Publishing Co., 1971.

Bois, Samuel J. *Art of Awareness.* Dubuque, Iowa : William C. Brown Co., 1966.

Bonny, Helen L. *Music and Your Mind.* New York: Harper and Row, 1973.

Bowman, William J. *Jogging.* New York: Grosset & Dunlap, 1967.

Bromley, D.B. *The Psychology of Human Aging.* Baltimore: Penguin Books, 1969.

Brotman, Herman H. "The Older Population : Some Facts We Should Know," unpublished paper, 1970.

Brown, Barbara B. *New Mind, New Body, Bio-Feedback: New Directions for the Mind.* New York: Harper and Row, Publishers, 1974.

Buck, Pearl S. "Creativity and the Aging American," *Psychosomatics,* VIII:4, Part 2, 1967, pp. 28-32.

Bultena, Gordon and Vivian Wood. "Leisure Orientation and Recreational Activities of Recreation Community Residents," *Journal of Leisure Research,* II:1, Winter, 1970, pp. 3-15.

Cain, Leonard D. "Age Status and Generational Phenomena," *Gerontologist,* VII:2, Part 1, June 1967, pp. 83-96.

California Recreation Commission. "Public Recreation and Parks in California," Sacramento: Documents Section, State Printing Office, 1957.

Cannon, W.B. *Wisdom of the Body.* New York: W.W. Norton & Co., 1932.

Caplan, Gerald. *Principles of Preventive Psychiatry.* New York: Basic Books, 1964.

Carlson, Reynolds E., Theodore R. Deppe, and Janet R. McClean. *Recreation in American Life.* Belmont, Ca.: Wadsworth Publishing Company, 1968.

Carp, Frances. "The Impact of Environment on Older People," *Gerontologist,* VII:1, March 1967, pp. 106-108, 135.

Cattell, Raymond B. "The Nature and Measurement of Anxiety," *Scientific American,* CVIII:3, 1963, pp. 96-104.

Chaiklin, Harris (Ed.). *Marian Chace: Her Papers.* Columbia, Md.: American Dance Therapy Association, 1975.

Clark, Margaret M. "The Anthropology of Aging: A New Area for Studies of Culture and Personality," in *Middle Age and Aging,* ed. Bernice L. Neugarten. Chicago: University of Chicago Press, 1968, pp. 433-443.

Comfort, Alex. "Can Life Be Prolonged? Should Life Be Prolonged?" Center Report III, The Center for the Study of Democratic Institutions, Santa Barbara, Ca., pp. 17-18, October 1970,

Cooper, Kenneth H., M.D. *Aerobics.* New York: J. B. Lippincott, 1968.

Corbett, Margaret Darst. *How to Improve Your Eyes.* Los Angeles: Willing Publishing Co., 1944.

Cratty, J. B. *Movement Behavior and Motor Learning.* Philadelphia: Lea and Febiger, 1964.

Cummings, Elaine et al. "Disengagement: A Tentative Theory of Aging," *Sociometry,* XXIII:1, March 1960, pp. 23-35.

Cummings, Elaine and W. E. Henry. *Growing Old.* New York: Basic Books, 1961.

de Beauvoir, Simone. *Coming of Age.* New York: G. P. Putnam & Sons, 1972.

De Cecco, John P. *The Psychology of Learning and Instruction: Educational Psychology.* Englewood Cliffs, N.J.: Prentice-Hall, Inc., 1968.

Devi, Indra. *Yoga.* Englewood Cliffs, N.J.: Prentice-Hall, Inc., 1959.

de Vries, Herbert A. *Physiological Effects of an Exercise Training Regimen, for*

Bibliography

Men Aged 52-88. University of Southern California Final Report to Administration on Aging. No date, pp. 34-36.

Dissertation Abstracts Index. Ann Arbor, Mi.: Subsidiary of Xerox Corporation, 5 volumes, 1965-1969.

Dowd, David J. "An Investigation of Some Social Factors Related to the Psychological Well-Being of the Elderly." Unpublished thesis, University of North Carolina, 1970.

Durkheim, Emile. *Suicide.* Glencoe, Ill.: The Free Press, 1951.

Ellfeldt, Lois, Ph.D. and Charles Leroy Lowman, M.D.,F.A.C.S. *Exercises for the Mature Adult.* Springfield, Ill.: Charles C. Thomas, 1973.

Erikson, Erik H. *Childhood and Society,* 2nd ed., rev. and enlarged. New York: W. W. Norton & Co., 1963.

——————. Identity, Youth and Crisis. New York: W. W. Norton & Co., 1968.

Exton-Smith; A.N. *Medical Problems of Old Age.* Bristol, England: John Wright and Sons, Ltd., 1955.

Feldenkrais, Moshe. *Awareness Through Movement: Health Exercise For Personal Growth.* New York: Harper & Row, Publishers, 1972.

Feng, Gia-Fu and Jerome Kirk. *T'ai Chi—A Way of Centering.* London: Collier-Macmillan, 1970.

Fisher, Seymour and Sidney E. Cleveland. *Body Image and Personality.* New York: Dover Publications, Inc. 1968.

French, J. D. "The Reticular Formation," *Scientific American,* Vol. 196, May 1957, p. 54.

Freud, Sigmund. *Beyond the Pleasure Principle.* Trans. and newly ed. by James Strachey. New York: Liveright Publishing Corp., 1961.

Garnet, Eva D. "Geriatric-Calesthenics," *Retirement Center Management,* March/April 1966, pp. 30, 37.

——————. *Theory and Philosophy of Geriatric-Calesthenics.* Los Angeles, California: Prepared for Teacher-Training Program funded by the Manpower Development and Training Agency (MDTA), 1963.

Goldfarb, Alvin I. Interview, by E.D.G., July 17, 1970.

Goldstein, Kurt. *The Organism: A Holistic Approach to Biology.* Derived from *Pathological Data in Man.* New York: American Book Co., 1939.

Gordon, Gilbert S. and Cynthia Vaughan. *The Clinical Management of Osteoporosis.* Acton, Mass.: Publishing Sciences Group, Inc., 1976.

Graham, Martha. *Notebooks of Martha Graham.* New York: Harcourt Brace Jovanovich, 1973.

Hall, Calvin S. and Gardner Lindsey. *Theories of Personality.* New York: John Wiley and Sons, 1970.

Hall, J. Tillman, Ph.D. *Dance! A Complete Guide to Social, Folk and Square Dancing.* Belmont, Ca.: Wadsworth Publishing Co., 1963.

Havighurst, Robert J. "Research and Development Goals in Social Gerontology," *Gerontologist,* IX:4, Part 2, Winter, 1969, pp. 18-33.

Havighurst, Robert J., Bernice L. Neugarten, and Sheldon S. Tobin. "Disengagement and Patterns of Aging," in *Middle Age and Aging,* ed. Bernice L. Neugarten. Chicago: University of Chicago Press, 1968, pp. 161-177.

Hawkins, Alma. *Creating Through Dance.* Englewood Cliffs, N.J.: Prentice-Hall, Inc., 1965.

H'Doubler, Margaret N. *Dance.* Madison, Wi.: The University of Wisconsin Press, 1966.

Hebb, Donald O. *A Textbook of Psychology.* Philadelphia: W. B. Saunders Co., 1966.

Herman, Michael and Mary (Eds.). *Folk Dancer Magazine,* P.O. Box 201, Flushing Station, Long Island, N.Y.

Heron, Woodburn. "The Pathology of Boredom," *Scientific American,* Vol. 196, January 1957, pp. 52-56.

Hittleman, Richard. *Richard Hittleman's Yoga.* New York: Workman Publications, 1969.

Humphrey, Doris. *The Art of Making Dances.* New York: Grove Press, 1959.

Hunt, Valerie. "Neuromuscular Organization in Emotional States." *What Is Dance Therapy Really?* Proceedings of the Seventh Annual Conference, American Dance Therapy Association, Columbia, Md., 1972.

Isaacson, Robert L., Max L. Hutt, and Milton L. Blum. *Psychology: The Science of Behavior.* New York: Harper and Row, Publishers, 1965.

Jacobson, Edmund. *Biology of Emotions.* Springfield, Ill.: Charles C. Thomas, 1967.

—————. *Progressive Relaxation.* Chicago: University of Chicago Press, 1929.

James, William. *Psychology: The Briefer Course.* New York: Crowell-Collier Publishing Co., 1962.

Johnson, Harry J., M.D. *"Creative Walking" for Physical Fitness.* New York: Grosset & Dunlap, 1970.

Jourard, Sidney M. *The Transparent Self.* Princeton, N.J.: D. Van Nostrand Co., Inc., 1964.

Keelor, Richard. "Physical Fitness," *Aging,* No. 252, October 1975.

Kleemeier, Robert W. "Leisure and Disengagement in Retirement," *Gerontologist,* IV:4, December 1964, pp. 180-184.

Kramer, Charles H., M.D. and Jeannette L. Kramer. *Basic Principles of Developing Long Term Care: Developing a Therapeutic Community.* Springfield, Ill.: Charles C. Thomas, Publisher, 1976.

Laing, R.D. *The Divided Self.* New York: Penguin Books, 1959.

La Meri (Russell Meriwether Hughes). *Gesture Language of the Hindu Dance.* New York: Columbia University Press, 1942.

Bibliography

_____. *Spanish Dancing*. New York: A. S. Barnes Co., 1948.

Land, George T. *Grow or Die*. New York: Random House, 1973.

Latner, Joel. *The Gestalt Therapy Book*. New York: Julian Press, 1972.

Lawton, George, M.D. *Aging Successfully*. New York: Columbia University Press, 1956.

Lee, Robert. *Religion and Leisure in America*. New York: Abingdon Press, 1964.

Lemkau, Paul V. "Prevention in Psychiatry," *American Journal of Public Health*, LV:4, 1965.

Logan, Gene A. and Earl L. Wallis. *Figure Improvement and Body Conditioning Through Exercise*. Englewood Cliffs, N.J.: Prentice-Hall, Inc., 1964.

Londoner, Carroll A. "Survival Needs of the Aged: Implications for Program Planning," *Aging and Human Development*, II:2, May 1971.

Lowen, Alexander, M.D. *Language of the Body*. New York: Collier Books, 1958.

_____. *Betrayal of the Body*. New York, Macmillan & Co., 1969.

_____. *Depression and the Body*. Baltimore, Md.: Penguin Books, Inc., reprinted 1974.

Maddox, George L. "Disengagement Theory: A Critical Evaluation," *Gerontologist* IV:4, Part 1, June 1964, pp. 80-82.

Maisel, Edward (Ed.). *Resurrection of the Body (Alexander Method)*. New York: New York University Books, Inc., 1959.

Maisel, Edward. *T'ai Chi for Health*. New York: Holt, Rinehart and Winston, 1972.

Maltz, Maxwell, M.D. *Psycho-Cybernetics*. New York: Pocket Books, 1972.

Martin, Alexander R. "Leisure Time—A Basic Health Resource." Sacramento: California Recreation Commission, Publication No. 58-M-3, August 1958.

Martin, John. *The Dance*. New York: Tudor Publishing Co., 1946.

_____. *The Modern Dance*. Brooklyn, N.Y.: Dance Horizons, Inc. 1933.

Maslow, Abraham H. *Motivation and Personality*. New York: Harper and Row, Publishers, 1954.

_____. *Toward a Psychology of Being*. Princeton, N.J.: D. Van Nostrand Co., 1962.

May, Rollo. *Existential Psychology*. New York: Random House, reprinted 1969.

Mensendiek, Bess. *Look Better, Feel Better*. New York: Harper and Row, Publishers, 1954.

Miller, Norman P. and Duane M. Robinson. *The Leisure Age*. Belmont, Ca.: Wadsworth Publishing Co., 1967.

Miller, Stephen J. "The Social Dilemma of the Aging Leisure Participant," in *Middle Age and Aging*, ed. Bernice L. Neugarten. Chicago: University of Chicago Press, 1968, pp. 366-374.

Montagu, Ashley. *Touching: The Human Significance of the Skin.* New York: Harper and Row, Publishers (Perennial Library Edition), 1972.

More, Thomas. *Utopia.* New York: Washington Square Press, 4th printing, 1968.

Morehouse, Laurence E. and Leonard Gross. *Total Fitness in 30 Minutes a Week.* New York: Simon and Schuster, 1975.

Moruzzi, G. & H.W. Magoun. "Brain Stem Reticular Formation and Activation Of The EEG," *Electroencephalography and Neurophysiology,* I, 1941, pp. 455-473.

Murray, Frank S. and Judith Safferstone. "Pain Threshold and Tolerance of Right and Left Hands," *Journal of Comparative and Physiological Psychology,* LXXI:1, 1970.

National Center for Health. "Statistics Survey, May-June, 1974." Public Health Service Publication No. N 1000 Series 212, No. 6. Washington, D.C.: Government Printing Office. (Reviewed in *Gerontologist,* VII:3, Part I, September 1967, p. 187.)

National Council of Teachers of English. *Guidelines For Non-Sexist Use of Language.* Urbana, Ill.: National Council of Teachers of English, 1975.

"National Institute of Senior Centers Inaugurated at March Conference," *Aging,* May 1970, pp. 4-5.

National Recreation Workshop. "Recreation for Community Living," Chicago: The Athletic Institute, 1952.

Neugarten, Bernice L.(Ed.) *Middle Age and Aging, A Reader in Social Psychology.* Chicago: University of Chicago Press, 1968.

North, Marion. *Personality Assessment Through Movement.* Norwich, Suffolk, England: The Chaucer Press, 1972.

Olds, James. "Pleasure Centers in the Brain," in *Contemporary Psychology.* San Francisco: W.H. Freeman and Co., 1971.

Orcutt, Dorothy J. "Evaluative Criteria for Administrative Measurement of Recreation Programs for Senior Citizens." Unpublished dissertation, Colorado State College, 1968.

Ornstein, Robert E. *The Psychology of Consciousness.* San Francisco: W.H. Freeman and Co., 1972.

—————. *The Nature of Human Consciousness.* New York: Viking Press, 1973.

Parrington, Vernon L. *Maincurrents in American Thought.* Vol. I. New York: Harcourt, Brace and Co., 1930.

Patty, William L. and Louise Snyder Johnson. *Personality and Adjustment.* New York: McGraw Hill Book Co., 1953.

Pelletier, Kenneth R. *Mind as Healer Mind as Slayer: A Holistic Approach to Preventing Stress Disorders.* New York: Delta Books, 1977.

Peppard, Harold M. *Sight Without Glasses.* Garden City, N.Y.: Doubleday, 1959.

Bibliography

Perls, Fritz S. *In and Out of the Garbage Pail*. Lafayette, Ca.: Real People Press, 1969.

Perls, F., R. Hefferline, and P. Goodman. *Gestalt Therapy*. New York: Delta Books, 1965. (Paperback)

President's Council on Aging. *The Older American*. Washington, D.C.: Government Printing Office, 1963.

Pressey, Sidney and Alice D. Pressey. "Geniuses at 80, and Other Oldsters," *Gerontologist*, VII:3, Part I, September 1967, pp. 183-187.

"Quotations from the Commissioner," *Aging*, May 1970, p. 8.

Rathbone, J. L. and Valerie Hunt. *Corrective Physical Education*. Philadelphia: W. B. Saunders Co., 1965.

"Recreation and Parks in Los Angeles," Los Angeles: Public Relations Division, City Recreation and Parks Department, 1968.

Reich, Charles A. *The Greening of America*. New York: Bantam Books, Inc., 1971.

Riley, Matilda White. *Aging and Society. Vol. I: An Inventory of Research Findings*. New York: Russell Sage Foundation, 1968.

Rodney, Lynn S. *Administration of Public Recreation*. New York: Ronald Press Co., 1964.

Rogers, Carl. *On Becoming A Person*. Boston: Houghton Mifflin Co., 1961.

Rolf, Ida P. *Structural Integration*. New York: Ida P. Rolf, 11 Riverside Drive, 1963.

Roman, P. and P. Taietz. "Organizational Structure and Disengagement: The Emeritus Professor," *Gerontologist*, VII:3, Part I, September 1967, pp. 147-153.

Rose, Arnold M. "A Current Theoretical Issue in Gerontology," *Gerontologist*, IV:1, March 1964, pp. 46-50.

Rugg, Harold. *Imagination*. New York: Harper & Row, Publishers, 1963.

Schilder, Paul. *The Image and Appearance of the Human Body. Part III, the Sociology of Body Image*. New York: International Universities Press, 1950.

Schoop, Trudi, with Peggy Mitchell. *Won't You Join The Dance?* Palo Alto.: National Press Books, 1974.

Selye, Hans. *The Stress of Life*. New York: McGraw-Hill Book Co., 1956.

_____. *Stress Without Distress*. New York: J.B. Lippincott Co., 1974.

_____. "Explorers of Humankind." Lecture, June 1978, Los Angeles Convention Center.

"Senior Citizens Manual," County of Los Angeles Board of Supervisors, N. S. Johnson, Director, County Department of Parks and Recreation, n.d.

Shanas, Ethel. "Health and Adjustment in Retirement," *Gerontologist*, X:1, Part 2, Spring 1970, p. 17.

Shanas, Ethel et al. "The Psychology of Health," in *Middle Age and Aging*, ed. Bernice L. Neugarten. Chicago: University of Chicago Press, 1968, pp. 212-219.

151

Silberman, Linni (Ed.). *Dance Therapy Bibliography.* Columbia, Md.: American Dance Therapy Association, 1980.

Spring, Evelyn L. "Professional Preparation in Recreation: Undergraduate Education Pertinent to Leadership with Older Adults." Unpublished doctoral dissertation, University of Southern California, 1968.

Steiglitz, Edward J., M.D. *The Second Forty Years.* Philadelphia and New York: J.B. Lippincott Co., 1952.

Stone, Gregory P. "The Play of Little Children," *Quest,* Monograph IV, Spring Issue, April 1965, pp. 23-31.

Tague, Jean R. "Leisure-time Activities in Selected Nursing Homes." Unpublished doctoral dissertation, University of Southern California, 1968.

"Teaching Athletes to Breathe Properly." *The First Aider for Women.* II:3, Jan. 1975, p. 2.

Thompson, Richard F. *Foundations of Physiological Psychology.* New York: Harper and Row, Publishers, 1967.

Thompson, Richard F. (Ed.). "New Findings on Reticular Formation," in *Foundations of Physiological Psychology,* Moruzzi & Magoun. New York: Harper and Row, Publishers, 1967.

Tiger, Lionel. *Optimism: Biological Roots of Hope.* N.Y.: Simon and Schuster, Inc. 1979.

Toffler, Alvin. *Future Shock.* New York: Random House, 1970.

U.S. Department of Health, Education and Welfare, "The Practitioner and the Elderly," in *Working With Older People,* Vol. 1, 1969. Washington, D.C.: U.S. Department of Health, Education and Welfare, 1969.

Van Nort, William. "History of Aging in Connection with Leisure Time." Unpublished paper, Department of Recreation, California State College, Los Angeles, 1966.

Weinberg, Jack. "Mental Health in the Aged," in *Restorative Medicine in Geriatrics,* ed. Michael M. Dasco. Springfield, Ill.: Charles C. Thomas, 1963, pp. 259-274.

Wells, Kathrine. *Kinesiology: The Scientific Basis of Human Motion.* Philadelphia: W.B. Saunders Co., 1966.

Western Gerontological Society. "Summary of Proceedings of the 15th Annual Meeting, October 9-10, 1969," 785 Market St., San Francisco, Ca. 94103.

White House Conference on Aging. "Recommendations Compiled from Section Reports Presented at Final Plenary Session," Washington, D.C., January 9-12, 1962.

Williams, Jesse Feiring. *The Principles of Physical Education.* Philadelphia: W. B. Saunders Co., 1964.

Youmens, Grant E. "Some Perspectives on Disengagement Theory," *Gerontologist,* IX:4, Part 1, Winter 1969, pp. 254-258.

Zubek, J.P. (Ed.). *Sensory Deprivation: Fifteen Years of Research.* New York: Appleton-Century-Crofts, 1969.

Index

Activity coordinators and directors, *see* Therapeutic community

Adaptive energy, 53

Aesthetics, 63-64, 87, 130, 137

Aging, xi ff. *See also* Biological aging, Well-aging

Anxiety, 7, 16-17, 36-38, 46, 54, 58, 77, 79

Arthritis, 14-15, 110

Atrophy, xi, 8, 12, 38, 63, 109

Auditory sense, *see* Senses

Automatic (basic) movements, 10-14, 19-22. *See also* Movements

Balance, 11, 14, 16, 30, 36-38, 91, 107-108, 110, 112

Basic Position, 71, 81-82, 88, 96, 104-107, 109, 127

Bending, 14, 32, 51, 53, 62, 99

Billingsley, Jack, 121

Biofeedback, xi, 22, 54, 58, 113

Biological aging, 3, 8-9

Biological clock, 3

Body-awareness, 12-14, 32-35, 38, 57-58, 72-74, 84, 101, 107, 109, 113, 140: Body language, 32

Body-image, *see* Body-awareness, Kinesthetic sense, Muscular innervation, Sensory awareness

Bones, *see* Musculoskeletal system, Osteoporosis

Brain (right and left), *see* Body awareness, Holistic health, Sensorimotor circuit

Breathing, 9, 11, 17, 22-25, 29-30, 37, 39, 51-52, 57-58, 68, 76, 86, 89-90, 96-97, 108, 112-114, 116, 122, 127

Calisthenics, *see* Geriatric body dynamics, Physical education

Cardiovascular system, 3, 11, 22-23, 25, 40, 112

Cassette tapes, 71, 76, 85-86, 90, 117, 138-139, 143

Centering, 30, 33, 95-96, 113

Chace, Marian, 85

Chair exercise, 48, 53-54, 62-64, 70, 115-119, 128-134

Change, 4, 8, 17-18, 24, 28, 33, 38, 46, 58-61, 70, 77, 85, 101, 106-109, 113-114, 129, 140, 142

Chronic illness, 6-8, 22, 24-25, 36-39. *See also* Disease

Circulation (blood), 9, 11, 17, 22-25, 39, 62, 91, 99, 108, 112-113, 116, 122, 136

Climacteric, 38-39

Clothing, 117, 134-137

Co-contraction, *see* Contractions

Color, *see* Senses

Contractions, 50-51, 62, 73, 98-99, 101

Convalescent hospitals, 5, 8, 24-27, 39, 63, 110-111, 123-126, 134, 138, 141

Culture, *see* Paradoxes of aging

Dance therapy, 56. *See also* Movement therapy

Depression, 36-38, 40-41, 48, 57-58, 64, 111, 113

Discussion, 75, 79-80, 109-115

Disease, 8, 34, 39-41: Arteriosclerosis, 40; Atherosclerosis, 8, 40; Cancer, 40; Cardiovascular disease, 40; Diabetes, 40, 136; Heart attack, 40; Parkinson's disease, 40; Stroke, 40, 49. *See also* Arthritis, High blood pressure, Osteoporosis

Disorientation, *see* Sensory deprivation

Distress, 8, 17, 33, 36-38, 58, 63, 74

Education, *see* Learning, Teaching techniques

Effort, 32, 51-53, 71-72
Emotion, 35, 56ff. *See also* Holistic health
Empathy, 31, 33, 65, 68, 75, 101, 143
Energy, (physical and mental) 11, 33, 38, 46, 51-55, 58, 60, 65-66, 68, 71, 86, 93, 101-102, 108, 123, 141, 143
Equilibrium, *see* Balance
Eustress, 8-9, 36-38
Exercise, 12ff.
Exercise Manual, 71, 82, 90, 104, 107, 139, 143
Exhilaration, 31, 36-39, 41, 48, 60, 63, 67-68, 118, 139, 141
Expressiveness (physical, self-, and verbal), 31, 48, 55-56, 66-67, 75, 86, 88-91, 101, 108, 112
Exteroceptors, *see* Senses

Falling, 16, 32, 50, 107
Feeling, *see* Sensory awareness
Food, *see* Nutrition

Geriatric Body Dynamics, 39, 41, 45ff.
Geriatric Calisthenics, *see* Geriatric Body Dynamics
Gerontology, 3
Gestalt Psychology, 30, 35, 139
Graham, Martha, 51
Gravity, 16, 32, 50-51, 53, 101
Grounding, 30, 33, 113
Group dynamics, 65-69, 102-103
Group therapy, *see* Geriatric Body Dynamics

Habit, 12-13, 18, 46, 69, 107
Hallucination, *see* Sensory deprivation
Health, 5-9, 11, 18, 22, 30, 33-35, 38, 46, 56, 59, 63, 67, 70, 102, 110, 116, 135, 139-141
Heterostasis, 8-9
High blood pressure, 34, 40, 114
Holistic health, xi, 24, 33-35, 69, 111-114, 139, 141
Homeostasis, 8-9, 18, 36-38, 46
Humor, 45, 67-68, 79, 85, 102, 113

Humphrey, Doris, 50-51
Hypertension, *see* High blood pressure

Imagery, xi, 32, 52, 89, 93, 111
Imagination painting, 75, 89-91
Innervation, *see* Muscular innervation
Intellect, *see* Mind
Intonation, 75-76, 85
Isometric contraction, *see* Contractions

Joints, *see* Musculoskeletal system

Kinesthetic sense, ix-xii, 29-30, 33, 41, 48-50, 57, 64, 75, 91-92, 100-101, 108, 122

Laughter, 47-48, 65, 67, 75, 79, 102
Learning, 12-13, 59ff.
Let go, 30-32, 96, 100
Long, John, Dr., 122

Manual instruction, 75, 83-85, 101, 130
Martin, John, 51
Medicare, 5
Memory, 29, 33, 49-50, 60, 86, 91, 100, 110, 113
Menopause, *see* Climacteric
Mental illness, 4-5, 7-9, 40
Mental set, 34ff. *See also* Holistic health
Mind (intellect), 28 ff. *See also* Holistic health
"Mirror me," 75-76, 80-81, 116, 130
Motivation (physiological and psychological), 36, 45-47, 55, 60, 65, 68-69, 72, 83, 102, 109, 117, 129
Motor skill, 107-109
Movement-readiness, xi ff.
Movement therapy, xi ff.
Movements: Axial (torso), 28; Head, 28; Pendular (arm or leg), 28; Percussive, 85; Succession, 51; Sustained, 85
Muscles, *see* Musculoskeletal system

Muscular innervation, 35, 72-74, 76-77, 81-82, 87-88, 104, 107-108, 128

Musculoskeletal system, 12, 14, 16-17, 20-21, 24, 28-31, 34, 50-52, 57-58, 62, 73-74, 76, 87, 98-99, 101-102, 107, 112-114, 122, 128

Music, 75, 85-88, 118, 126

Needs, *see* Six S's
Nervous system, 9, 29, 35, 48, 58, 74, 94, 101, 112, 114, 116
Nutrition, 5, 11, 110, 114, 126

Olfactory sense, *see* Senses
Optimism, 68-69
Osteoporosis, 38-40

Pain, xi, 6, 10-11, 14-16, 38, 47-48, 52, 54, 57-58, 63, 73, 97-100, 122, 142
Pairing, 75, 84, 93-101, 130, 132-134
Paradoxes of aging, 15-18, 61
Perception, *see* Pain, Sensory awareness
Physical education, 56, 78
Placebo effect, 70, 100
Pleasure, xi, 33, 36-39, 46-48, 58, 62-64, 72-73, 86, 93, 102
Position of Relaxation, 95
Postural set, *see* Posture
Posture, 16-18, 74, 104-108
Psychosomatic continuum, 36-41
Publicity, 119-126
Pull, 30-31, 33, 112
Push, 30-31, 33, 56, 112

Reality ("Here and now," Reality orientation), 27, 30, 124
Rebound, *see* Gravity
Recreation, 12, 15-16, 24, 108, 122, 140
Relaxation, 29-30, 32-33, 47-48, 50-52, 54, 57-58, 62, 74, 79, 89-90, 100-102, 108, 112, 114-115, 123, 126, 128: Differential and progressive, 52. *See also* Let go, Position of Relaxation

Respiration, Respiratory system, *see* Breathing
Restoration therapy, 46
Retirement, 3-6, 13, 15, 19, 21, 24-25, 46, 59, 116, 140
Retirement homes, 6-7, 21-22, 24, 54, 63, 110, 121-123, 126, 141
Rhythm (movement and musical), 10-12, 16, 45, 49-50, 52-53, 56, 64, 67-68, 75-76, 87-90, 92-93, 99, 103, 111, 115, 118, 127: Rhythmic verbalization, 76
Ritual, 64, 69-71, 115, 136

"Say it," 75-77
Self-awareness, 73ff.
Self-image, xi ff.
Semantics, 77-78
Senescence, 3, 5, 6, 11, 35-41, 45, 77, 109, 112
Senility, 3-5, 7-8, 36-41, 112
Senior citizen centers, 7, 24, 54, 63, 110, 126, 141
Senses, xi-xii, 27-29, 40-41, 46-50, 52, 71, 73-74, 80, 86, 91-94, 108, 110, 112, 114, 123-124, 139
Sensori-motor circuit, 58, 74
Sensory awareness, xi, 28-33, 48, 56, 71, 73, 91-94, 107-109, 114
Sensory deprivation, 40-41, 48, 111, 124
Sensory stimulation, 27, 46-50, 73-74, 91, 124
"Show me," 75-76, 81-82, 91, 101
Six S's (supplement, stimulation, safety, support, significance, satisfaction), 46-50
Skeletal system, *see* Musculoskeletal system
Stress, 4, 7, 8-9, 30, 33-34, 36-38, 45, 53-54, 57-58, 63, 87, 107, 112, 123
Stress theory, 7-9
Stretching, 14, 32, 51, 53, 56, 58, 62, 99, 101, 105, 116
Suspension, *see* Gravity
Swinging, 31, 50-51, 56, 68, 103, 118, 127. *See also* Gravity
Synergistic action, 51, 62, 99

Teaching techniques, 45ff.

Tension, 28, 33, 38-39, 46, 51-52, 57-58, 62, 71, 74, 94, 97-102, 110, 112, 114, 122: Residual tension, 52, 74, 101

Therapeutic community, 5, 22, 24-27, 119-126

Touch, 27, 29, 40-41, 49-50, 58, 72-73, 75, 80-85, 91, 93-101, 110, 112-113, 124

Visual sense, *see* Senses

Vitality, xii, 35-38, 41, 50, 56, 64, 76, 80, 128, 140-142

Well-aging, 6-7, 22, 24-25, 36

Wheelchairs, 24, 27, 49, 53, 130, 132

Work ethic, *see* Retirement